Seminars in Respiratory Disease

Peter A. Petroff, MD

Clinical Professor, Texas State University

2025 Edition

Copyright 2024

Dedicated to the faculty of the

Respiratory Therapy Department of

Texas State University.

Index

Introduction	vii
How to use this book	ix

Part One

Seminar 1:	COPD	1
Seminar 2:	Asthma	15
Seminar 3:	Pneumonia	31
Seminar 4:	Pulmonary Arterial Disease	51
Seminar 5:	ARDS	69
Seminar 6:	Congestive Heart Failure	83

Part Two

Seminar 7:	Diffuse Parenchymal Lung Disease	99
Seminar 8:	Neurologic Disease	115
Seminar 9:	Cancer of the Lung	133
Seminar 10:	Diseases of the Pleura	147
Seminar 11:	Cystic Fibrosis	163
Seminar 12:	Disorders of Sleep	181
INDEX		197

Introduction

"Seminars in Respiratory Disease" is the last course respiratory therapy students complete before graduation. I believe that is as it should be. It is the only course that "brings it all together." The course combines a clinical case with anatomy, physiology, and diagnostics including radiographs, arterial blood gases and pulmonary function testing, as well as the treatment of the case patient especially the role of the respiratory therapist. No other university level course provides this degree of integration.

In addition, the seminar course demands the aspiring graduate prepare a written report and perform an oral presentation relating to the particular case under consideration. The student must be ready to stand in front of his fellow students and the course professor and present his ideas about the case and, just as importantly, be ready to defend them. This is no mean task.

The reward for the student is the knowledge that he or she is ready to be accepted into the medical community. He or she will be able to communicate with doctors, nurses, and the administration about what is important for the care of the patient and what is important for his respiratory therapy department. Communication is the key to the care of the severely ill patient.

How to Use This Book

Each "seminar" begins with a brief overview of a particular disease that can affect the respiratory system. This is followed by three cases which include major aspects of a patient's history, physical findings, diagnostic testing, and treatment. Following the cases studies is the key points the student must include in his or her presentation and a discussion of these major points. Lastly there are topics for "minor" papers to be prepared by the students in the class who just listened to the presentation.

The student will begin his paper and presentation with the case history. The patient is always the fulcrum of the paper and presentation. He or she will then, using the key points, create his or her own understanding of what is going on with the patient. The student must become a detective and answer several questions. Was the patient's history and physical typical for the disease diagnosed by the treating physician? Was the diagnosis correct? Should other tests have been done? Was the treatment appropriate? Could any other illness account for the findings? The student then must present an overview of the disease including its anatomy, physiology, pathology, and treatment.

The major paper should have a front sheet, identifying the subject, the topic or the paper, the author of the paper and the class. An abstract should follow. In general, the abstract is about a page in length and gives a substantial review of the findings of the paper. Next, there is an introduction. This should ask the question, "Why is this important." The whole paper follows. Finally, there is a conclusion which answers the question posed in the introduction.

The "minor" paper is a two to three-page report created by the students who listen to the presentation. Often, it is simply a reformation of the high points of the presentation, but ideally it is independent research of the topic under discussion. The minor paper replaces the multiple-choice question testing normally used for grading. The use of the "minor" papers encourages the listening student to take notes about the presentation, read the notes, and create his or her own paper. Thus, learning is approached on several levels, not just memorizing facts presented during the seminar supplemented by a hopefully good guess on an examination.

The minor paper certainly creates additional work for the class instructor. Each paper must be graded and corrected. But the student learns from the corrections. When I first began using the system it was clear to me that the students, even though they were in the fourth year of university, had written very few, if any, papers. Grammar, spelling, and word choice were not of the level needed for accurate in-hospital communication between respiratory therapists, nurses, and doctors. Most of what they wrote was "TV Speak." While this style of writing or speaking might be appropriate at home or with friends at a restaurant or bar, it could never be an appropriate form of communication for the hospital chart or for running a respiratory care department.

When I teach the course, I grade the students as follows. Each student presents two major seminars, each presentation and paper worth a total of thirty points. The presentation (15 pts) is graded on the following:

1. The student's appearance,
2. The students use of slides. Does he or she simply read the Power Point slides or does he or she uses them more as a guide to his or her presentation?
3. The student's interrelationship with the listeners. Does he or she answer questions well and does he or she involve the students in the discussion?
4. The content of the material presented.

The paper (15 pts) is graded on its structure:

1. Does it have a face sheet, abstract, an effective introduction, a good body of information and a concluding paragraph which addresses the points raised in the introduction?
2. Are the spelling and grammar correct?
3. Are there adequate references?
4. Are the references in the appropriate format?

There should be ten minor papers, each paper worth 4 points. They are graded on:

1. Structure of the paper. Does it have a good beginning, body of information, and conclusion?
2. How is the spelling, grammar, and word-choice,?
3. Was there any independent research, or original ideas presented with appropriate references?

There are a handful of reference materials that I highly recommend. **Linz's Comprehensive Respiratory Disease**, edited by Sindee Karpel and Anthony Linz and published by Jones and Bartlett Learning, is the most thorough and current (published in 2019) textbook directed to the respiratory therapy student. It has numerous charts and drawings which help clarify the text. Much of it is well-written though at times the text gets bogged down in details.

Up To Date is a medical journal aimed primarily at physicians. However, the text is quite readable, and the respiratory therapy student should be readily able to comprehend it. There are more than 6000 articles which are constantly updated and thus are quite current. It is published by Wolters Kluwer. More than 1.7 million physicians in more than 150 countries use the journal regularly. In addition, it is available from the Texas State University (and probably most universities) free of charge to students.

The best medical textbook is, of course, **Harrison's Principles of Internal Medicine** which is now in its 21st edition, published in 2022. It is edited by Jameson, Fauci, Kasper, Hauser, Longo and Loscalzo and published by McGraw Hill Education. The index alone is more than 214 pages! The text is more than 3500 pages. Harrison's gives an overview of each disease, a description of the physiology and pathology, a differential diagnosis as well as the current therapy. In addition, diseases that are related to the primary diagnosis are discussed in detail. The cost of the book is a problem for any student ($155 at Amazon), but the book should be available in most university libraries.

Principles of Pulmonary Medicine by Weinberger, Cockrill and Mandell and published by Elsevier and now in its seventh edition (2023) is by far the best text of pulmonary disease or respiratory therapists. It is comprehensive yet, because it is so well-written, it is quite approachable. Rarely can you say that reading a textbook is enjoyable but reading "Principles" is! It is a book so well written that you can't put down. In addition, if the student purchases the print-book (about eighty dollars), he or she will be able to upload the e-book for free!

Lastly, I must give a plug for my own book, **Lecture Notes, Anatomy and Physiology for the Respiratory Therapy Student**. The textbook is updated regularly and covers the major diseases the respiratory therapy is likely to encounter. It is available at Amazon for a pittance.

One

Chronic Obstructive Lung Disease

Chronic obstructive lungs disease (COPD) encompasses four quite different diseases: emphysema, chronic bronchitis, bronchiectasis, and asthma. They all differ physiologically. Emphysema is due to the loss of the elastic supporting structure of the lung. Chronic bronchitis is due to thickening of the lining of the small and large airways caused by inflammation. Bronchiectasis results from severe, unremitting infection of the bronchi culminating in irreparable destruction of the airways. Lastly, asthma is due to inflammation of the bronchi causing the smooth muscle of the airways to become "twitchy."

Yet all the diseases share a common property. They are all primarily caused by inflammation. The inflammation may have different causes and produce different effects and the inflammatory pathway may not be exactly the same, but inflammation is the common denominator.

In addition, all diseases called COPD affect the airways predominantly. They all cause narrowing or obstruction of the airway, although in each case, the mechanism is different. For example, emphysema causes obstruction because the loss of airway support during exhalation allows airways to collapse whereas chronic bronchitis causes airway obstruction because the lumen of the airway is markedly narrowed by inflammation and pus.

Most people view COPD as a "catch-all" for chronic bronchitis and emphysema since the two diseases often coexist and, in general, share the same major causation of cigarettes and air pollution. If we limit COPD to just those two disorders, it is still the third most common cause of death at present in the USA and soon will be the third most common cause of death in the world. More than 65,000,000 people throughout the world including 12,000,000 Americans suffer from the disorder. More than 3,000,000 die from the disease each year. Yet, to a very large extent, it is a preventable disease.

Peter A. Petroff, MD

Case Presentations

1.

Dr. Walker was giving a demonstration of new office-based pulmonary testing devices at her large multispecialty clinic to a group of family practice physicians. After showing them how the machines work, how they can be used in their practices, and how important pulmonary testing is, she asked for a volunteer from the group to be her "guinea pig." Dr. Everett, a family doctor, stepped forward. He was 34 years old, of average height at 5'10" and average weight at 175 lbs. Dr. Walker entered the data on the machine's keypad. She then asked Dr. Everett to perform a forced vital capacity. After a few seconds, the results were posted on the machine's LED screen. Dr. Walker turned towards Dr. Everett, "Do you smoke?" Dr. Everett answered as he stared at the computer screen, "Never. Not even one cigarette."

Dr. Walker showed the results to Dr. Everett. His forced vital capacity (FVC) was normal at 4.5 liters, but his forced expiratory volume in one second (FEV1) was only 2.5 liters and his FEV1/FVC ratio was very low at 55%, normal being greater than 75%. Moreover, the flow volume curve was "scooped out," a finding consistent with chronic obstructive lung disease. Dr. Walker asked Dr. Everett to see her later that day in her office.

Dr. Everett returned that afternoon. He said he had no symptoms at all. He works 10-12 hours a day. He plays tennis twice a week. He never smoked, in fact, no one in his family ever smoked. He did grow up on a farm but never did any farm work. His past history was totally unremarkable. He doesn't drink, doesn't take any medicines, has no drug allergies, has never been hospitalized and never had any surgery. His parents are living and well. His father still works on the farm.

Dr. Walker did a simple examination. Dr. Everett's O2 saturation was 95%. His pulse and blood pressure were normal. His examination was totally normal except for his lungs. Dr. Walker noted that his chest appeared to be hyperinflated with a tympanic percussion note over all the lung fields. His breath sounds were diminished symmetrically.

Dr. Walker then had Dr. Everett do complete pulmonary function testing using a "body box." The total lung capacity (TLC) was 115% of predicted; the residual volume (RV) was 125% of predicted. The FVC and FEV1 were as before. The diffusing capacity was markedly reduced at 75% of predicted. There was no change in values after a bronchodilator was given.

Dr. Walker told Dr. Everett that he probably had emphysema. She asked him to get a chest X-ray and some blood tests which he did. The following morning, he returned to her office.

The chest x-ray showed hyperinflation with widened rib spacing and flattened diaphragms. The heart shadow was narrow. The hilar shadows were enlarged consistent with mild cor pulmonale. There was pruning of the pulmonary vessels which was most pronounced at the lung bases.

The level of alpha-1-antitrypsin was 25; normal is more than 200. Dr. Walker had ordered a genetic profile which showed that Dr. Everett had two ZZ genes consistent with alpha-1-antitrypsin deficiency. His blood count and chemistry panel were normal.

The two physicians reviewed the data together. Dr. Everett had a heritable cause of emphysema. While he could take replacement therapy with intravenous Alpha-1-antitrypsin shots given twice monthly, as of this moment there was not much evidence of its efficacy in people who were asymptomatic. Dr. Everett asked about having children. Dr. Walker suggested testing Dr. Everett's wife. It turned out Dr. Everett's wife was ZM. In other words, Dr. Walker said she was a carrier with one normal gene and one abnormal gene. Dr. Walker told him that his children would either be carriers of the disease like his wife or have the disease like he did. She recommended that his children should be tested as well.

Dr. Walker suggested that rather than start replacement therapy now, she would recheck Dr. Everett's pulmonary function in six months and see if there is any change. He would get a pneumonia shot and continue to get his flu shot annually.

2.

Sam H. is a 67-year-old male who comes to the outpatient clinic complaining about his cough. He states he has coughed for years, in fact, more than twenty years. But in the last week the cough has gotten worse, and his sputum has changed to a greenish color with specks of blood. He states emphatically that he is not short of breath. He has no history of pneumonia. In fact, he has no history of any lung disease.

He tells the doctor he smokes a little more than a pack a day. He has smoked for 45 years. He smokes "Kools," a mentholated cigarette because it does not irritate his throat as much. He has no history of lung disease. He states emphatically, "Cigarettes never hurt anyone." In fact, if he doesn't smoke when he gets up, his cough is worse.

Sam's past medical history (PMH) was reviewed. He doesn't drink. He takes an over-the-counter sleep medicine. He is not allergic to any medicine. He has never had any surgery or been in the hospital. He works as a machinist at a factory that makes specialized auto parts. He always wears a mask while working. His mother died of lung cancer. His father died of colon cancer. His brother, two years older than Sam, just had a heart attack.

Sam is 5'6" and weighs 200 lbs. He has an obvious productive cough. He doesn't appear to be short of breath, at least at rest but his lips are bluish. His O2 saturation is 86% on room air. His BP was 156/86. His pulse was 86. He is afebrile.

Outside of the mild bluish discoloration of his lips, the examination of his head and neck exam is normal. His lungs show a few expiratory wheezes and coarse crackles which clear after coughing. The breath sounds are decreased. His heart is normal in size to percussion. The heart sounds normal.

There are no murmurs. The liver is slightly enlarged. There is 1 + pedal edema. The pulses in his feet are absent.

The doctor tells Sam he may have pneumonia on top of his COPD. After noting the absent pulses in Sam's feet, he tells Sam he likely has peripheral vascular disease as well. The doctor sends Sam for an immediate chest x-ray to make sure whether there is or is not a pneumonia.

The chest x-ray showed a right lower lobe pneumonia but was otherwise normal.

The doctor admits Sam to the hospital. He orders arterial blood gases, a sputum gram stain and culture, a CBC, and a chemistry profile. He begins Sam on oxygen at 2 l/min via a nasal cannula, IV fluids, IV Zithromax, albuterol nebulizer treatments every four hours and low molecular weight heparin. The heparin is given subcutaneously in order to prevent clotting.

The blood gases were done on room air:

the pO2 was 54

the pCO2 was 58

the pH was 7.24

the HCO3 was 28

The WBC was high at 12,000 with a shift to the left (more neutrophils); the gram stain of the sputum showed gram positive intracellular diplococci consistent with S. pneumoniae infection; the chemistry profile was normal.

Over the next twenty-four hours, Sam felt better. His cough improved and the color of the phlegm returned to its more typical grey-yellow color. The blood gases were repeated on oxygen.

The pO2 was 78

the pCO2 was 48

the pH was 7.45

the HCO3 was 26

The following morning the blood gases were checked on room air. Sam's pO2 was now 62 with an O2 Saturation of 88%. The doctor recommended that Sam go home with oxygen and an albuterol inhaler four times a day. Sam promised he would quit smoking. He was scheduled to return to the doctor's office in two weeks.

Sam returned to the doctor's office two weeks later. He had stopped smoking. His O2 saturation on room air was now up to 94% and the doctor said he could stop using the O2. He continued the albuterol as needed and asked Sam to return for a follow-up chest x-ray and pulmonary function testing in another month.

The chest radiograph was now normal. The pulmonary function testing was consistent with moderate COPD:

FVC	80% of predicted
FEV1	45% of predicted
FEV1/FVC	56% of predicted
TLC	100% of predicted
RV	125% of predicted
DCO	normal

There were no changes in the pulmonary function tests following the use of a bronchodilator.

Sam was allowed to return to work and agreed to see the doctor in six months. He was to use an albuterol inhaler as needed. He also agreed to get a screening minimal dose CAT scan of the chest in 3 months to check for an early lung cancer.

3.

Mary A. is a very pleasant elderly woman who comes to the outpatient clinic because of a cough she has had for years. She says, "Every time I cough, I lose a friend. They all think I have Tuberculosis. I have no one to play bridge with anymore."

Mary states she is 78 years old. She is thin, amiable, and dressed appropriately for her age. Her cough is indeed frightening. Every time she coughs, she coughs up a handful of thick green phlegm. Mary says that she coughs up a half cup of phlegm a day. Recently she has been getting short of breath with exertion, but she is still able to take care of herself. She has coughed up blood from time to time but has no fever or night sweats. She has not lost any weight although her appetite is, "Not as good as it used to be." She has no history of asthma or pneumonia. She has never smoked. No one in her family ever had anything like this. She lives alone. Her husband died more than 15 years ago. She worked as a secretary for a law firm for nearly forty-five years until she retired 6 years ago. She has a comfortable retirement income.

She is 5 feet tall. She weighs 85 lbs. Her BP and Pulse are normal. Her O2 saturation is 96% on room air at rest. She is afebrile. Her examination is normal save for the examination of her lungs which show diffuse expiratory crackles as well as fine inspiratory crackles over the right lower lobe.

The doctor orders an immediate chest radiograph (PAL).

The chest x-ray shows not only a right lower lobe pneumonia but also diffuse interstitial changes with patchy atelectasis. The radiologist also mentions the presence of "tram lines" and suggests Mary has bronchiectasis.

The doctor decides to treat Mary as an outpatient because her pulse rate and O2 saturation are reasonable. He will treat her with a "Z-pack" (Zithromycin). He will also have her get outpatient laboratory studies including a CBC, Chemistry profile, sputum gram stain and culture, sputum smear and culture for tuberculosis, immunoglobulin panel (IgG, IgM, IgA, and IgE), a sweat test, and a test for HIV (Human Immunovirus). *Why did the doctor get all these blood tests?*

Mary returns in three days. She is definitely feeling better, and her cough is better as well. The doctor reviews the findings with her. The laboratory tests were all normal. The sputum grew S. pneumoniae which is the likely cause of her pneumonia. But although the smear for tuberculosis was positive, she did not have M. tuberculosis; rather she had Mycobacterium avium, an atypical tuberculosis organism.

The doctor explained she had Lady Windermere's Syndrome, named after a character in a play by the British playwright and humorist, Oscar Wilde. He sent Mary for a High-Resolution CAT scan which showed right middle lobe bronchiectasis with some cylindrical bronchiectasis in both lower lobes. He also sent her for another sputum test, this time to learn which antibiotics could be best used to treat her atypical tuberculosis organism.

The doctor recommended triple therapy consisting of Zithromax, three times a week, Ethambutol and Rifampin. She would need to take the medications for a year. In addition, she needed to do chest physical therapy, including both a chest vibrating device (The Vest) and postural drainage, twice a day. She was also to use a nebulizer with albuterol four times a day. He administered a pneumonia vaccine and advised her to get a flu shot every year. He would follow her monthly with a chemistry profile to make sure her liver tests were normal. He also sent her to an eye doctor to have her retina examined. She would also need an eye exam every three months while taking the Ethambutol.

Background for the presentations

The three cases present three different patients with three different types of COPD. The first patient has emphysema due to Alpha-1-antitrypsin deficiency; the second patient has chronic bronchitis due to smoking, and the third patient has bronchiectasis due to an infection with Mycobacterium avium. They demonstrate the range of symptoms, signs, and physical findings the disorder labeled COPD may present with.

Important points

1. Pulmonary function testing should be done in all patients with suspected COPD.
2. The key finding on the PFT is the reduced FEV1/FVC ratio. The FEV1 and the FVC can be reduced in restrictive disease, but the FEV1/FVC ratio will be normal.
3. Alpha-1-antitrypsin deficiency is found not only in patients with emphysema but also in patients with chronic bronchitis, bronchiectasis and even a few patients with asthma. All patients with emphysema, chronic bronchitis and bronchiectasis should be tested for the disorder as should patients with treatment-resistant asthma.
4. The diffusing capacity is helpful. It is abnormal in emphysema and, in fact, may be the only test that is abnormal in that condition. It is normal in chronic bronchitis and asthma.
5. A good family history is always important.
6. Getting the patient to quit smoking must be the first line of therapy.

7. All patients with COPD need to get a one-time pneumonia vaccination as well as the flu vaccine yearly. They should also get the RSV (Respiratory Syncytial Virus) vaccine as well
8. Emphysema, chronic bronchitis, bronchiectasis, and asthma, no matter how different they seem, are all inflammatory conditions.

Discussion

All chronic obstructive lung diseases are characterized by airway obstruction whether the disease process is in the airway itself or in the surrounding parenchyma. Both emphysema and chronic bronchitis show a decreased FEV1 and a decreased forced vital capacity. In addition, all obstructive diseases must have an FEV1/FVC ratio of less than 0.7. The normal ratio is 0.7 or more. Diseases involving the parenchyma, such as pneumonia or pulmonary fibrosis, can have both a decreased FEV1 and FVC but the FEV1/FVC ratio is normal.

Chronic bronchitis is defined **clinically** as the presence of a cough for at least three months of the year for at least two years in a row while emphysema is defined **pathologically**, or more realistically, by a high-resolution CAT scan of the chest, characterized by the destruction of the lung parenchyma resulting in the enlargement of the air spaces. Bronchiectasis is defined **clinically** by unique clinical and radiological patterns. The patient coughs up two or more ounces of phlegm daily while the chest radiograph shows "tramlines" or patchy infiltrates. Asthma is defined **physiologically** by the presence of significant "reversibility" of the airway obstruction. The airways of the asthmatic are "twitchy."

While all COPD is worsened by cigarette smoking, both active and passive, both emphysema and chronic bronchitis are largely caused by cigarette abuse. At the present time there are more than 35,000,000 smokers in the United States, but the prevalence of smoking has decreased dramatically over the last fifty years. Sadly, there are now as many women smokers as men smokers. As of 2022, there were more than 3 million Americans with COPD.

Most individuals start smoking while in their mid to late teens. Nevertheless, only twenty percent of people who smoke get COPD. Why some smokers get COPD while some don't is still under study.

The effect of "vaping" both in getting people addicted to tobacco and in helping people to quit smoking cigarettes is still largely debatable. E-cigarettes are battery powered electronic devices which deliver heated nicotine and propylene glycol or glycerol into the lungs. The spray may also contain tin, lead, nickel, and arsenic. When e-cigarettes were first introduced in China in about 2003, they were intended to help people quit smoking but now there is more evidence than ever that they get young teens addicted. In 2016, about 3% of Americans overall were current users, but among high school students in 2018, 21% were current users. While the use of e-cigarettes is safer than conventional cigarettes, there is also some early evidence that they can cause a chronic cough as well as asthma and perhaps cancer of the lung as well. The main concern is that e-cigarettes will result in increased nicotine addiction as teenage users grow up. This year, the FDA proposed banning Juul vaping devices entirely. Mentholated and flavored tobacco has already been banned.

Tobacco smoke impinges on the small airways where it damages the mucosal lining of the bronchiole by penetrating into the submucosa of the airway setting off an inflammatory reaction. The basic concept is that there is balance between proteinases and anti-proteinases in the lung tissue. Proteinases are needed to destroy invaders but if left unchecked they will begin to destroy the lung tissue itself, especially the elastic supporting structure of the lung. The lung makes anti-proteinases to keep the proteinases in check. Tobacco smoke triggers the inflammatory reaction drawing neutrophils packed with proteinases into the small airways. The proteinases overwhelm the anti-proteinases resulting in damage to the small airways, and ultimately in fibrosis of the airways, as well as in the nearby alveoli. Both chronic bronchitis and emphysema are the result. A recent study suggests that vaping aggravates the effects of smoking.

A secondary cause of both emphysema and bronchitis is genetic, specifically alpha-1-antitrypsin deficiency. Alpha-1-antitrypsin is manufactured in the liver and secreted into the blood where it travels to the lung. It is an anti-protease and like other anti-proteases it is important in turning off the proteases produced by inflammation before they destroy the lung. If it is absent the lung will be damaged by the proteinases. The gene for the Alpha-1-antitrypsin protein is a codominant gene. The normal gene is labeled M. If you have two M genes, as most of us do, you will have about 200 mg/deciliter of the antitrypsin in the blood. There are two abnormal genes, S and Z. The presence of two S genes will result in a mild decrease in the antitrypsin level but if the patient has two Z genes there will be near total absence of the antitrypsin. He or she will have exceptionally low levels of the antitrypsin, between 20 and 30 mg/deciliter. A carrier of the genetic defect with one Z gene and one normal M gene or a patient who has a genetic makeup of SZ will have intermediate levels of the alpha-1-antitrypsin of about 70 mg/deciliter and will likely either have no symptoms or suffer from chronic bronchitis if he or she is a smoker.

A much less common cause of COPD is air pollution. In developing countries peat is still used for indoor cooking. In addition, SO2 (sulfur dioxide) and NO2 (nitrogen dioxide) are present in the exhaust of both gasoline and diesel-powered cars. Both chemicals form acids, sulfuric acid, and nitric acid, respectively, when combined with water.

Chronic bronchitis is characterized by hypertrophy of the submucosal glands, inflammation of the medial (middle) layer of the bronchial wall and a profusion of the goblet cells in the epithelium resulting in thickening of the bronchial wall and the production of copious amounts of mucous. The thickened bronchial wall blocks the small airways resulting in areas of the lung with low ventilation to perfusion ratios or "relative shunting." The ventilation-perfusion inequality causes hypoxemia and hypercarbia.

The typical patient with chronic bronchitis is the "blue bloater." Most often the patient is mildly to moderately obese. He or she complains of a cough but not shortness of breath, at least early on in the course of the disease. They usually visit the doctor because while they have had their cough for years, maybe a decade or two, it is clearly getting worse and now is interfering with their activities. They want the doctor to get rid of their cough. When they are seen, they are often cyanotic. When they sit down, they plunge or slump into the chair. They don't sit in the tripod position like the patient with emphysema. They do not struggle to breathe. The breath sounds are decreased with a prolonged expiratory phase and there may be inspiratory and expiratory coarse crackles which sometimes clear after coughing. Occasionally there are wheezes. Their heart may be slightly enlarged in size to percussion. The second sound may be increased in the pulmonic area which is to the left of the sternum at the 2nd interspace. Their liver may be enlarged, and they may have some edema. They are in the "fifty-fifty-fifty club." Their pO_2 is 50, their pCO_2 is 50 and their hematocrit is 50.

Their pulmonary function testing generally shows a normal total lung capacity (TLC) because the elastic recoil of the lung and the patient's muscle strength are not impaired. The Functional Residual Capacity (FRC) is normal or slightly increased. Because the airways are narrowed and close earlier in expiration, the Residual Volume (RV) is increased resulting in an increased RV/TLC ratio. They trap air. Of course, they have a decreased FEV1 and FEV1/FVC ratio.

Emphysema is characterized by destruction of the alveolar walls and its surrounding capillary network resulting in the presence of large non-functioning blebs and bullae. This results in increased dead-space ventilation or areas of high ventilation/low perfusion. You would expect the carbon dioxide to rise in such a circumstance. But the patient compensates by hyperventilating. Their blood gases remain normal, except during an exacerbation. The loss of the elastic supporting structure makes the small airways more collapsible during exhalation. The collapsing airways is what causes the obstruction.

The patient with emphysema, then, is the "pink puffer." They are thin. They burn a lot of energy breathing, as much as 4000 calories a day in fact. Their main complaint is shortness of breath. They fight for air. When they sit in a chair, they sit in the tripod position. Their arms lean on the sidearms of the chair, or rest on the doctor's desk or their elbows rest on their thighs. They lean forward. The skin over their thighs may be thickened and darkened from irritation caused by their elbows. They are and appear air hungry. If they have quit smoking, they do not even cough. But their blood gases are normal!

The patients with emphysema have decreased elastic recoil, their compliance curve is steeper, and because of that their TLC is increased. In addition, the airways have lost their elastic support and collapse with exhalation resulting in a markedly increased RV. The lung compliance curve shifts to the left, altering the balance between the chest wall and the lung, which causes the FRC to increase as well.

There are two types of emphysema which sometimes causes confusion. If the emphysema involves alveoli throughout the lung, from the respiratory bronchioles to the alveolar ducts and alveoli, then it is labeled as panlobular. On the other hand, centrilobular emphysema involves the alveoli arising only from the respiratory ducts. Panlobular emphysema usually involves the lower lobes and is the type of emphysema found in alpha-1-antitrypsin deficiency. Centrilobular emphysema is typically found in smokers in association with chronic bronchitis.

Both the patients with chronic bronchitis and emphysema develop cor pulmonale but the mechanisms are quite different. In the patient with chronic bronchitis, the pulmonary hypertension and subsequent cor pulmonale is due to hypoxemia and to a less degree hypercarbia, both of which cause vasospasm. When the hypoxia and hypercarbia improve, the pulmonary hypertension improves and the cor pulmonale resolves. They often go in and out of cor pulmonale for years and years. On the other hand, the patient with emphysema has lost not only the elastic support to his airway but also the capillary bed. This results in ever increasing pulmonary artery pressure and pulmonary hypertension leading to irreversible cor pulmonale. Since the problem is anatomic and not physiologic, it is not correctable with oxygen. When the patient with emphysema develops cor pulmonale he or she is at the end of the line and generally dies within a few months.

Treatment for patients with mild disease includes bronchodilators including B adrenergic agents such as albuterol as well as anticholinergic agents such as ipratropium. Long-acting B adrenergic or anticholinergic agents can be added for more severe disease. During acute exacerbations oral or intravenous steroids are often used. Certainly, for the patient with mainly chronic bronchitis, an inhaled steroid will likely be helpful and should be used with bronchodilators. A new agent, a phosphodiesterase-4-inhibitor, Roflumilast, which is given orally, decreases inflammation and relaxes the airway smooth muscle.

Daily or thrice weekly azithromycin, a macrolide antibiotic, is also used for some patients with chronic bronchitis. Macrolides are not only antibiotics, but they also have anti-inflammatory properties.

Therapy with oxygen is important and should not be overlooked in these patients. If the patient has a resting O2 saturation of less than 88% or a paO2 of less than 55, the patient will generally benefit from oxygen therapy used around the clock or at least more than 15 hours a day. If the paO2 falls between 55 and 60, but the patient also had findings of cor pulmonale or polycythemia (hematocrit > 55%), he or she will also likely benefit from oxygen. The O2 saturation should also be checked at night. Some patients only desaturate at night. If the nocturnal O2 saturation is less than 88% then the patient should receive nocturnal O2. Patients who only desaturate with exercise generally are not helped by oxygen.

The patient who is a true pink puffer has little options. These patients do not respond to bronchodilators and have only minimal response to steroids. Nevertheless, these agents should be used, along with antibiotics, during an exacerbation of their disease. If the patient is deficient in alpha-1-antitrypsin then consideration should be given to intravenous replacement of the antitrypsin. As of this moment, even though the genetic abnormality is well described, "gene therapy" (replacing the abnormal gene with a normal gene) is not yet an option.

Both pulmonary rehabilitation and exercise strengthening are good options for both the "blue bloater" and "pink puffer" and all the shades in between. In addition, they should get the pneumonia vaccine, annual influenza vaccinations and the RSV vaccine. Needless to say, smoking must stop if they are still smokers.

Surgery for patient with COPD is limited. A few patients may benefit from "lung reduction surgery" but these patients are truly few and far between. In the patient with end-stage emphysema lung transplantation is an option. Life expectancy after a transplant has improved dramatically in the last ten years.

"Lung reduction surgery" involves removing parts of the lung in order to improve the pulmonary mechanics. It has been used in the past to treat patients with "bullous emphysema." These patients' bullae so large that the normal lung becomes compressed. Removing the large bullae allows the normal lung to expand. Bullous emphysema is an unusual form of emphysema often seen in young men. In the last two decades lung reduction surgery has also been done in patients with more typical emphysema. The initial results were positive, but over time it has become clear that not all patients benefit from the surgery. "Patient selection" is of paramount importance. At first, the surgery was done by physically removing lung tissue but recently, less invasive surgeries have become available.

How does lung volume reduction therapy work? In patients with emphysema, the loss of the elastic supporting structure of the lung causes a shift to the left of the pulmonary compliance curve (pressure-volume curve) resulting in hyperinflation as well as air trapping. The FRC increases as does the TLC. As the disease progresses, the lungs function near the top of the compliance curve, which is flattened meaning there is less change in lung volume for any given change in pressure. This results in an increased work of breathing. In addition, because of the hyperinflation, the inspiratory muscle fibers of the diaphragm and chest wall are shortened and less effective. Because emphysema is characterized as a "patchy" disease, the emphysematous areas compress the normal areas causing atelectasis. Lung reduction surgery increases the elastic recoil of the lung resulting in a lower FRC and TLC. In addition, lowering the TLC makes the thorax more normal in size and shape allowing the respiratory muscles to function better.

Patients who had a more homogenous emphysema or a markedly decreased diffusing capacity did poorly with lung reduction surgery, as did patients who had heart disease, pulmonary hypertension, the chronic use of steroids, or who had need for more than 6 liters minute of oxygen. Patients with primarily upper lobe disease did best.

Recently endobronchial valve implantation or "valve therapy" has been developed. This consists of implanting a one-way valve into a bronchus. The valve allows air and mucous to flow out but not in. Over time, this causes the lung distal to the valve to collapse reducing hyperinflation. Studies to date show a significant reduction in TLC and RV as well as an increase in FEV1, six-minute walk distance and quality of life. The most common complication was pneumothorax. But a few patients died.

Very recently, non-invasive ventilation has been tried for patients with chronic respiratory failure. Several studies suggest that it is helpful in improving life expectancy and reducing hospitalizations in patients with COPD and a high carbon dioxide level. Most of the therapy has been done with BiPAP. The patient must use the BiPAP at least four hours a night. The goal is to reduce the elevated PaCO2 by 20% to nearly normal levels. The treatment is approved by Medicare.

The GOLD (The Global Initiative for Obstructive Lung Disease) standards for the diagnosis, management, and prevention of COPD are updated yearly. The most recent update was published in November of 2023 for the 2024 year. These guidelines should be thoroughly reviewed by the student of respiratory disease. The most important points of the 2024 guidelines include the importance of the FEV1/FVC ratio in establishing the diagnosis of COPD. In addition, they include a new category of patients with "preCOPD" who have a history of respiratory symptoms and findings of abnormal pulmonary function testing with a normal FEV1/FVC ratio. These patients are defined to as having "PRISm" or "preserved ratio impaired spirometry." The GOLD guidelines also suggest that anyone with dyspnea, cough, wheezing, a history of recurrent pulmonary infections or a history of risk factors, such as smoking, should be evaluated for COPD. The guidelines also classify patients with an FEV1/FVC ratio of less than 0.7 into different degrees of severity. GOLD 1 is "mild" and the FEV1 is more than 80%; GOPD 2 is "moderate" and the FEV1 is between 50 and 80%; GOLD 3 is "severe" with an FEV1 between 30 and 50%; GOLD 4 is "very severe" with an FEV1 of less than 30%. In the past, treatment was largely based on this severity scale. In the last few years, the guidelines for treatment have become much more complicated.

Two symptom scales have been added. The first is the "modified Medical Research Council" or mMRC scale of dyspnea. There are five levels from Grade 0, "dyspnea only with severe exercise" to Grade 4, "I am too short of breath to leave the house" or "I get short of breath dressing or undressing." Recently, a "multidimensional" questionnaire has also been added called the CAT or "COPD assessment test." The test asks the patient to evaluate his own degrees of cough, shortness of breath, chest discomfort, confidence or feeling or well-being, and energy level. The scores on each question range from 0 to 5. Thus, a patient can have a score from 0 to 40. Lastly, the blood eosinophil count must be measured. Normal is less than 150 cells/microliter of blood, but the guidelines use a "cut-off" of 100.

The guidelines stress that the number one therapy is to encourage the patient to quit smoking, but the use of vaccines and avoiding other risk factors is also stressed.

Treatment is now based on:

1. Is there a history of exacerbations? If the patient has had two moderate exacerbations or one exacerbation that results in hospitalization, he or she should be placed in "group E" and should be treated with an LABA (long-acting b-adrenergic agent) combined with a LAMA (long-acting muscarinic agent). If the patient has an elevated eosinophil count, inhaled corticosteroids ICS) should be added. Thus, most patients will be on triple therapy.
2. If the patient has one or less exacerbations then they will fall into either group A or B depending on their symptomatology based on the mMRC or the CAT. If the mMRC is one or less and the CAT score is less than 10, then the patient falls into

group A should be treated with a bronchodilator of some type. If the patient has an mMRC of 2 or higher or a CAT of more than 10, they fall into group B and should be treated with a combination of LABA and LAMA.

Bronchiectasis shares some features with chronic bronchitis in that the primary feature of both diseases is a "cough." But in the patient with bronchiectasis the cough is productive of more than two ounces of phlegm a day. The disorder is defined as irreversible destruction of the bronchi and bronchioles due to inflammation and subsequent scarring of the bronchial tubes. In general, it is due to infection and is found throughout the lungs, but in a few cases, it can be localized if it is caused by an obstructed airway, perhaps due to an inhaled peanut, a tumor or even inspissated mucus, with infection superimposed on the blocked airway. In the past, measles and pertussis were the main causes of the disease. Nowadays the major player worldwide is Mycobacterium tuberculosis. Another type of tuberculosis infection is caused by the organism Mycobacterium avium complex (MAC). This is an "atypical" Mycobacterium which can't be transferred from person to person which causes localized disease in the immunocompetent patient, usually bronchiectasis involving the right middle lobe known as Lady Windermere's Syndrome, or a generalized disease in the immunocompromised patient such as the patient who has the HIV.

Bronchiectasis can also be caused by immune-incompetency such as in the patient with an immunoglobulin deficiency, most commonly, hypogammaglobinemia, or a patient with dysfunction of the cilia lining the bronchi which impairs the ability of the mucociliary ladder to clear secretions. One example of this is Kartagener Syndrome which is characterized by the presence of situs inversus in addition to the ciliary dysfunction causing both inflammation of the sinuses and bronchiectasis.

Pathologically the airways of the lungs are markedly abnormal. Some are cylindrically dilated, some are irregularly dilated, and some are just large sacs. Some of these sacs are filled with pus. Lymphocytes and neutrophils pack the mucosa and submucosa of the airways. Scarring of the bronchiole tubes is universal. The arteries supplying the bronchial tubes are larger and because of the overlying inflammation and mucosal ulceration sometimes bleed profusely if they are biopsied.

The most common cause of bronchiectasis is Cystic Fibrosis (CF), but non-CF bronchiectasis is becoming more common in patients even in their sixties. The patient's main concern is their cough which often costs them their friends. The sputum is copious and purulent and sometimes bloody. Two, four, six, or even eight ounces a day of phlegm are not uncommon. Examination of the patient reveals extensive wheezing, as well as coarse expiratory crackles, and sometimes even fine inspiratory crackles, over the diseased areas of the lung. Clubbing is common. The patient's chest radiograph is abnormal. There are increased interstitial markings, "tramlines" which represents the thickened walls of a dilated bronchus, and "signet rings" which are bronchi with thickened walls partially filled with pus. The high-resolution CAT scan of the lungs is diagnostic. The test is mandatory in that it provides not only a definitive diagnosis but also reveals the extent of the disease which is important in deciding on therapy.

Blood gases will show mild to moderate hypoxemia with mild respiratory alkalosis early on. As the disease worsens or during exacerbations there is often a respiratory acidosis.

Sputum culture grows Pseudomonas aeruginosa and Staphylococcus aureus. However most acute exacerbations are due to S. pneumoniae and Hemophilus influenza and respond well to Zithromycin. Of interest, the microbiome (the organisms normally present in the lungs) is usually characterized as having several distinct species. In a patient with bronchiectasis the diversity of organisms is decreased, and one or two organisms take over completely. Pseudomonas, Enterobacteriaceae, and Stenotrophomonas can cause severe disease with Pseudomonas the deadliest. Hemophilus and Streptococcus, while common, are not associated with severe disease. The FEV1 decreases fastest in patients with Pseudomonas.

The treatment is directed both at the infection and the copious secretions. Inhaled tobramycin (Tobi) is often used to help control infections. A new formulation of tobramycin, using a dry powder will soon be available. If the patient has M. avium, then multiple antitubercular agents are needed. The antibiotics are chosen based on the sensitivity of the organism. Postural drainage and percussion as well as the use of a "pneumatic vibrating chest wall vest" or a "flutter valve" are especially helpful and must form the backbone of therapy. B adrenergic agents promote the mucociliary function and are effective. Inhaled corticosteroids and the chronic use of a macrolide antibiotic may help the underlying inflammation and should be considered.

Surgery is reserved for patients who have severe life-threatening hemoptysis or who have very localized disease. One common location for bronchiectasis is the right middle lobe and surgery is often successful in patients with the right middle lobe syndrome. For most patients, bronchiectasis involves more than a single lobe of the lung and surgery, except for a lung transplant, is not going to be of value.

Suggestions for minor papers

1. What are the effects of vaping on the airways?
2. Compare the PFTs in patients with emphysema and chronic bronchitis.
3. How does emphysema cause airway narrowing? Compare that to chronic bronchitis.
4. What is the Kartagener syndrome?
5. What is cor pulmonale?
6. How do B adrenergic agents work?
7. How do anticholinergic or anti-muscarinic agents work?
8. What are the different causes of bronchiectasis?
9. Discuss Alpha-1-antitrypsin deficiency.
10. Discuss lung reduction surgery and lung transplantation.
11. Discuss NIV (non-invasive ventilation) usage in patients with respiratory failure.

Two

Asthma

Asthma is defined as an obstructive airway disease which is at least partially reversible. For many, this implies that asthma is essentially a disease of "twitchy airways." But the root cause of asthma is airway inflammation. The inflammation may be caused by atopy or allergy, infection, a dysfunctional inflammatory pathway, or causes still unknown. But inflammation is what makes the airways hyper-reactive. Thus, the treatment for asthma must be directed at both the reactive airways and at the underlying inflammation.

Asthma is divided into two large camps. Extrinsic asthma (T2 HI or Th2 asthma) is "allergic" asthma. It is most often seen in children and teenagers who often have a family history of allergies. It is often associated with other allergic or atopic conditions such as eczema or allergic rhinitis. The disease is characterized by markedly increased immunoglobulin E (IgE) and by the presence of large numbers of eosinophils. Intrinsic asthma (T2 LO or Th1 asthma), on the other hand, is a disease of older adults and is associated primarily with inflammation. While IgE is normal, the gamma globulin (IgG) is often increased. The disease may be related to airborne pollutants such as sulfur dioxide, formaldehyde, nitrogen dioxide or particulate matter. The disease may be work related. TDI or toluene diisocyanate is a widely used industrial chemical which can cause asthma. Asthma can even be related to exposure to certain viruses, especially RSV, and bacteria. It can be due to a fungus colonizing the bronchial lining (Allergic Broncho-Pulmonary Aspergillosis or ABPA). It can also be due to dysfunctional leukotriene response as in "Aspirin Allergy."

The treatment of asthma has become more and more effective. In addition to bronchodilators such as B-adrenergic agents, anticholinergic (anti-muscarinic) agents, and theophylline which is a diasterase inhibitor, we now have anti-inflammatory medications including inhaled corticosteroids, antibodies which bind directly to immunoglobulin E, and antibodies which bind to the leukotrienes responsible for causing the inflammatory reaction directly blocking the asthma pathway. Inhaled phospho-diasterase inhibitors will soon be making their appearance. The horizon is becoming brighter for the effective treatment of even the most refractory asthma.

Peter A. Petroff, MD

Case Presentations

1.

Rory is a twelve-year old young man who has had asthma since he was an infant. He came to the emergency room with a severe asthma attack which began the morning of admission.

According to his mother, he had a normal delivery and development until the age of three when he began having frequent "viruses" characterized by coughing and wheezing. His pediatrician treated him for infection after infection but after several attacks the mother demanded that he be sent to a pediatric pulmonologist. The pediatric pulmonologist did several tests including a CBC, eosinophil test, a test for immunoglobulins, a sweat test for cystic fibrosis and an airway oscillation test to measure airway resistance. He found mild eczema on examination of the child's skin.

The blood count showed an increased eosinophil count at 14%. The total eosinophil count was also increased. The IgG and IgM were normal, but the IgE was markedly elevated. The sweat test was normal. The airway oscillation test showed increased airways resistance which responded to bronchodilators.

Based on the testing, the pediatric pulmonologist diagnosed Rory with asthma and began him on a long-acting B-adrenergic agent. The doctor hoped to avoid using inhaled steroids because of their potential effect on the child's growth. He also gave the young boy a rescue inhaler. A nurse instructed the mother and Rory in their use. With practice and the use of a "spacer" the young lad was able to master the inhalers.

Rory did well for several years but in the last year he took a turn for the worse. He began waking with asthma nearly every night. The pulmonologist was quite concerned. He asked the mother if anything had changed. The mother noted that Rory was spending time at a friend's house, and that when he came home from visiting his friend, his eyes were watery and red, and he was wheezing. He had to use his inhaler several times to get relief. The doctor asked Rory about this. Rory said that his friend had a Persian cat. The doctor then did allergy testing. Rory was 4+ allergic to cats but surprisingly little else. The doctor told Rory's mother that Rory could not visit his friend's house. His friend could visit Rory after school at Rory's house instead. Rory improved and was back on the long-acting B adrenergic (LABA) agent alone.

The morning of admission, Rory had to go to his friend's house to get some papers for a school project. The friend's father, a smoker, then drove the two to school. After about an hour at school, Rory began to wheeze. Initially the wheezing responded to the rescue bronchodilator but by afternoon Rory was severely short of breath. His mother left work, picked him up at school, and took him to the emergency room.

Rory did not smoke, Vape, or use illicit drugs. His only medications were the LABA and rescue inhaler. He was not allergic to any medications. He had never had surgery and never had been in hospital before. His mother had asthma as a child.

Rory's height and weight were in the 50th percentile for his age. His blood pressure was 96/52; his pulse was 126; he was afebrile.

Examination of the head and neck showed red watery eyes and mild cyanosis of the lips.

Examination of the lungs showed decreased chest wall movement, moderate tympani on percussion, and the breath sounds were markedly diminished though there were scattered fine expiratory and inspiratory wheezes.

The cardiac examination was normal as was the abdominal exam and the examination of the extremities.

The doctor ordered a CBC and ABGs and began Rory on continuous albuterol nebulization. He also ordered IV fluids and intravenous cortisone (40 mg IV Solumedrol stat and every six hour). He began Rory on oxygen at two liters per minute per nasal cannula.

The blood count was normal. The pO2 was 64 (on room air), the pCO2 was 28, the pH was 7.5 and the HCO3 was 24.

After an hour, Rory felt better. The doctor re-examined him. When he listened to Rory's lungs, he heard diffuse inspiratory and expiratory wheezes. He also heard breath sounds. He admitted Rory to the hospital.

The Albuterol nebulization treatments were decreased to every four hours and as needed. Intravenous cortisone was continued every six hours. By the following morning, the wheezing was nearly gone, and Rory was "ready to go home," at least according to Rory. The doctor advised Rory and his mom to avoid any exposure to cats at all. Rory was to resume his LABA. He could use his inhaler every four hours today and then go back to using it as needed. The doctor also continued oral cortisone. Rory was to take 40 mg a day of prednisone for four days then stop. He was to see the doctor in a week.

2.

Kathy M. is a 36-year-old woman who comes to the clinic because she is short of breath. She has been short of breath for more than six months. At first it was mild, and it only occurred a day or two every week but in the last month the shortness of breath has been every day and is to the point that she can only walk a hundred feet before she has to rest.

She tells the doctor she has had a cough which she describes as a dry, irritating cough. She has also noticed that she is wheezing. She never had asthma, but she imagines she sounds like an asthmatic. She has not had any chest pain. She has never seen a doctor before.

The doctor reviews her past medical history. She has never smoked. She does not drink. She is taking a birth control pill. Sometimes she takes a Tylenol or Motrin for arthritis. She is not allergic to any medications. She has never had any surgery or been admitted to hospital. Her mother and father died from cancer. There is no history of asthma in the family.

Her examination reveals audible wheezing. Her BP is 145/85. Her pulse is 86. Her temperature is normal. She is 5'4" and weighs 145 lbs.

Examination of the head and neck is normal. Her lungs show decreased breath sounds with grade two wheezing, both inspiratory and expiratory, which is polyphonic. Her heart sounds are normal. Her abdominal and extremity exam is normal.

The doctor orders a chest radiograph and pulmonary function studies.

The chest x-ray shows slight bibasilar interstitial changes. They are minimal. The radiologist describes them as "dirty lungs."

The PFTs show (as percent of predicted):

	Prebronchodilator	Postbronchodilator
FVC	75%	82%
FEV1	45%	60% (a 33% improvement)
MMF	30%	45% (a 50% improvement)
TLC	119%	
RV	108%	
DCO	100%	

The patient returns. The doctor tells she has asthma but nothing else to worry about. She is shocked. She has never had asthma. No one in her family has had asthma.

The doctor then asks her, "Your symptoms began once a week?" She answers, "Yes, always on Monday when I went back to work. The wheezing would get worse during the week, but I never had problems on the weekend. I was really good when I went on vacation."

The doctor asks, "What kind of work do you do?" Kathy M answers, "I work with circuit boards. I fuse the large chips to the board." The doctor then asks, "Do you wear a mask?" Kathy M answers thoughtfully, "No, we were never told we needed to wear a mask."

The doctor then arranges to have Kathy do a peak flow measurement on Monday before she goes to work and then repeat again at her lunch hour. Sure enough, the peak flow falls more than 25% between the two readings.

The doctor concludes she has work related asthma. He begins her on an albuterol metered dose inhaler to use as needed, a long-acting B-adrenergic agent, an inhaled steroid, and a short course (5 days) of prednisone. She is to return in a week. She is not to go to work.

Kathy M. returns in a week. She is much better but is still wheezing some. Her FEV1 is now 65% of predicted. The doctor tells her she has lung disease caused by the chemical *toluene diisocyanate*. He states she can no longer work at the same job. If she does so, she will eventually be totally disabled because of scarring in her lungs, a condition he calls pulmonary fibrosis.

3.

Shelly C. is a spritely young lady, 22 years of age, who is admitted to hospital with pneumonia. She states she has had asthma since she was 12. She always hoped to outgrow it but just never did. She uses a short-acting B adrenergic agent as a rescue inhaler, as well as an inhaler which includes both a long-acting beta-adrenergic agent (LABA) and a long acting anti-cholinergic or muscarinic agent (LAMA). She uses an inhaled steroid during flare-ups. She was doing well with no more than three nighttime awakenings a month until a week ago. Suddenly she developed wheezing that did not respond to her rescue inhaler, even when she used it every three hours, or to her inhaled steroid. She also had fever with mild chilliness and a cough productive of yellow phlegm. She says the phlegm was "disgusting." "It was so thick I could chew it."

In the emergency room, a chest radiograph was done which showed a right middle lobe infiltrate. The radiologist was concerned that there were "tramlines" and asked the emergency room physician if the patient might have bronchiectasis.

The patient was a never smoker or drinker. Her medications included only her sprays for asthma. She had no drug allergies, surgery, or medical admissions. Her parents were living and in good health. No one in the family had asthma.

Her exam showed a temperature of 102 degrees F, her blood pressure was 124/74, her pulse rate was 102, and her respiratory rate was 20. She was 5'2" and weight 106 lbs.

Examination of her head and neck was unremarkable.

Her lungs showed decreased breath sounds with grade two wheezing throughout. The wheezing was polyphonic. There were fine inspiratory crackles over the right middle lobe.

The rest of the exam was normal. She did not have any clubbing.

The emergency room physician called a pulmonologist to see Shelly. After speaking with Shelly and examining her, he ordered a sputum culture and gram stain, a blood culture, a sputum for fungi, a sputum for eosinophils, a blood count, an eosinophil count, a sweat test, and an immunoglobulin panel. Most of the tests would take a day or two to come back. The sweat test would have to be done as an outpatient at the Cystic Foundation Center.

He began her on nebulized albuterol every three hours, IV fluids, Solumedrol 40 mg every six hours, Zithromycin, and oxygen.

The next morning, she was feeling much better. Her fever was gone, and her cough was better. The wheezing was much less. There were still fine crackles over the middle lobe.

The blood count showed an increased WBC, but the neutrophils were only mildly increased. There were nearly 15% eosinophils. The eosinophil count was markedly elevated as was the IgE.

The gram stain and culture of the sputum showed only a mixed flora consistent with oral secretions.

The sputum for fungi grew an organism which turned out to be Aspergillosis fumigatus.

The patient's pneumonia resolved over the next four days She was discharged on her albuterol, combination LABA and LAMA inhaler and prednisone (an oral steroid) at 20 mg a day.

She was seen in the office a week later. Her sweat test was normal. Her chest radiograph now showed mild increased interstitial markings. The doctor told her she had "Allergic Aspergillosis."

The doctor continued her medications although he decreased the prednisone to 10 mg a day. He thought she would have to take the prednisone "for some time."

Background for the presentations

These three cases illustrate different aspects of asthma. The first patient has "extrinsic" or allergic asthma. He has a family history of asthma. He has a history of eczema. He has an increased IgE and eosinophil count. He has a known trigger for his asthma: cats. The second patient on the other hand has "intrinsic" asthma. She has new onset asthma even though she is in her mid-thirties. She has no prior history of asthma, no family history of asthma, and normal lab values for eosinophils. Her asthma is caused by a chemical she is exposed to at work. Treatment in this case **must be** total avoidance of the causative agent. The last patient has asthma due by colonization with the fungus aspergillosis. The aspergillosis is causing an allergic reaction resulting in her asthma. The fungus is not invading the lung; rather it resides on the surface of the bronchial tubes. The patient then develops an allergic response to the fungus. Treatment is often difficult requiring both antifungal agents and some form of cortisone. Some patients will require lifetime oral steroids.

Important points

1. Asthma can affect anyone at any age.
2. Asthma is an inflammatory disease which causes "twitchy airways."
3. Asthma is divided into two categories depending on the cause of the inflammation: allergic or non-allergic, "extrinsic" or "intrinsic." But this division is quite arbitrary. Extrinsic asthma can occur in adults as well as children. Intrinsic asthma can be due to extrinsic factors such as an infection with the Respiratory Syncytial Virus or Mycoplasma, chemicals in the environment, or other "extrinsic" factors. Because of that, most pulmonologists

refer to the phenotype as either Th2 or Th1 or T2 HI or T2 LO depending upon whether allergy is involved or not.
4. Treatment must be directed at both the inflammation and the bronchospasm.
5. Treatment of the bronchospasm involves either **increasing *cyclic AMP***, by increasing the enzyme *Adenyl cyclase* using B adrenergic agents or blocking the enzyme *phosphodiesterase* which breaks down cyclic AMP by using theophyllines or **inhibiting *cyclic GMP*** by blocking the enzyme Guanylyl cyclase with an anticholinergic agent.
6. Treatment of the inflammatory pathways involves the use of both oral and inhaled steroids as well as using antibodies which either inhibit the leukotriene system by binding to TSLP (Thymic stromal lymphopoietin) or to leukotriene 4, 5, or 13, or which bind directly to IgE.

Discussion

Asthma is one of the most ancient of diseases. There are references to "noisy breathing" in Chinese records dating back more than 4500 years ago. The Code of Hammurabi, written about half a millennium later, described patients who "panted with work." Hippocrates, about 2500 years ago, was the first person to actually use the term "asthma" which comes from the Greek word "aazein" which means "to inhale with a gaping mouth" or "to pant" to describe patients with lung disease. The Macedonian general Alexander the Greek, who lived in the third century BC, reported that the residents of India used an anticholinergic agent (stramonium) to help their breathing. Two hundred and fifty years later Pliny, a Roman, recommended the use of "ephedra" (an epinephrine like agent) as a treatment for asthma. In 100 AD Aretaeus of Cappadocia, a Greek doctor, gave the first true description of asthma. He stated that the symptoms of asthma included intermittent heaviness of the chest and difficulty breathing as well as a severe cough.

Asthma has a worldwide distribution. As of 2016, 4.3% of the world's population and 8.4% of Americans had asthma. In the United States 9.5% of children and 7.7% of adults had asthma. It is more common in boys (8.3% versus 6.7%) and in adult women (10.8% versus 6.5%). It is more prevalent in Black people compared to Caucasians, but the highest incidence is in the Puerto Rican population.

Between 100 and 150 million people around the world suffer from asthma. The disease kills more than 180,000 people annually. In Western Europe, the incidence of asthma has doubled in the last ten years. In the United States, the incidence has climbed 60% since the early 1980's and more than 5,000 Americans die each year from the disease. Asthma care costs more than 6 billion dollars a year. In April of 2022, more than 25 million Americans had asthma according to the CDC.

Thus, asthma is a severe, world-wide, and costly disease whose frequency is increasing rapidly. It is primarily an inflammatory condition which causes the airways to become hyper-responsive to many different stimuli. Several factors, both inherited and acquired, contribute to the risk of developing asthma. Perhaps, hereditary factors are the most important, at least among children and young adults who are said to have extrinsic asthma. These patients often have a family history of asthma, a history of other allergic conditions such as eczema and allergic rhinitis, allergies demonstrated by skin testing and increased levels of IgE and blood eosinophils. Yet studies have never shown a unique gene responsible for either allergy or asthma. Likely this is due to the fact that several different genes are involved. Recently, a gene that promotes Interleuken 4 has been found. People who have an abnormal form of the gene have an increased incidence of mild (but not severe) asthma.

Environmental causes include exposure to allergens which are agents that provoke an asthmatic or allergic response in childhood as well as exposure to maternal smoking. Certain viral infections may increase the risk of asthma while still others may decrease the risk; this is the *hygiene hypothesis*. The incidence of asthma in Eastern Europe increased markedly after the fall of the Soviet Union. At first, this was thought to be due to better recognition of asthma, but the evidence suggests that the increase was real.

The allergic inflammatory pathways of asthma are slowly becoming better understood. When an allergen, bacteria, virus, fungus, or other foreign body is inhaled, it is trapped in the muco-ciliary blanket covering the airways. The epithelium contains "Alarmins" which are interleukin-like chemicals. Three types are currently known: TSLP, IL 33, and IL 25. These chemicals then trigger the asthmatic pathway. TSLP is **thymic stromal lymphopoietin** and is primarily involved in allergic or T2 HI asthma. It signals the Th 2 cell which then turn on IL 5, IL 4, and IL 13. IL 4 turns on the B cells which produce IgE. IL 13 and IL 5 activate eosinophils and basophils. The Ige produced by the B cells binds to the IgE receptor sites on mast cells. In addition, IL 13 also activates more Th2 cells, amplifying the reaction.

After the first exposure to an allergen, when the allergic individual is again exposed to the allergen, whether pollen, house dust, or cat dander, a dendritic cell or "antigen-presenting cell" identifies the allergen as "foreign" and presents the antigenic material to the Alarmins which activate the Th2 (helper 2 lymphocyte) which then release IL-4 and IL-13 and activates the IgE secreting B lymphocytes which become plasma cells. The plasma cell IgE binds to the IgE receptor sites on the mast cells and even the circulating basophils resulting in the release of a host of mediators. Some of these mediators cause bronchoconstriction directly. These include histamine, bradykinin, serotonin, and direct acting leukotrienes, which are derived from arachidonic acid by way of the lipoxygenase pathway and include LTC4, LTD4, and LTE4. The eosinophils also release toxins which cause epithelial damage. Growth factors are also produced which result in "remodeling" of the airways by causing smooth muscle hyperplasia and fibrosis or scarring of the airways. Interestingly, nitric oxide, a potent vasodilator, is also released during the inflammation.

We often compare allergic asthma or extrinsic asthma with non-allergic asthma or intrinsic asthma. Recently these groupings have been expanded into *phenotypes*. The extrinsic asthmatic has become the **allergic phenotype or "T2 HI"**, while the intrinsic asthmatic also called **"T2 LO"** has a different inflammatory pathway. In intrinsic asthma, the alarmins trigger Th 0 which then activates IL 4, IL 12, and IL 6. The IL6 stimulates the production of Th2, Th1, and Th17.

The classic T2 LO patient has normal levels of eosinophils, low IgE, and may have increased IgG. The patient tends to be older, without an allergic history. In addition, the patient does not respond well to steroids whereas the T2 HI patient is steroid responsive.

It turns out that asthma probably involves a spectrum from T2 LO to T2 HI. Some of the intermediate patients may have tissue eosinophil and sinusitis without evidence of allergies. This type of asthma is called the **eosinophilic phenotype.** Another type is the obese patient with asthma has become the **obesity-related phenotype**. The obesity-related asthmatic involves a different inflammatory pathway involving the helper 1, T lymphocyte (Th1) pathway rather than the Th2 pathway seen in most other types of asthma.

One very interesting type of allergic or T2 HI asthma is "Thunderstorm Asthma." Some patients with allergic asthma experience an exacerbation after a thunderstorm. It appears the pollen grains become waterlogged and explode releasing an avalanche of pollen. Patients who experience exacerbations with thunderstorms should avoid being outside during the pollen season.

Pathological findings of the bronchial tube in asthmatic patients reveal a host of findings. The lumen of the airway is markedly narrowed and filled with mucous. There may be Curschmann's spirals which are microscopic casts of the ducts of the mucous glands. There is damage to the epithelial lining of the airway along with edema of the entire bronchial wall, hypertrophy of the smooth muscle layer of the bronchus and infiltration of the mucosa with inflammatory cells such as eosinophils and lymphocytes. There is also hypertrophy of mucous secreting glands and a marked increase in the number of goblet cells. The basement membrane is thickened as well.

Because not all of the bronchi are involved to the same extent, ventilation is not distributed evenly throughout the lungs. However, perfusion remains largely intact. This results in ventilation/perfusion inequality. In areas that have low ventilation with preserved perfusion, a relative shunt develops which causes the pO2 to fall. The patient compensates by breathing faster and thus the pCO2 is decreases and the arterial blood gases, at least acutely, are characterized by a respiratory alkalosis. If the disease process becomes very severe the ventilation/perfusion inequality will worsen, the pCO2 will rise, and a respiratory acidosis will occur.

Clinically, asthmatics can present with many different symptoms. The patient typically presents with "shortness of breath," but some present with "tightness in the chest," while others present with a "cough after I work out," and still others present with "a cough that always wakes me in the middle of the night." Most patients will describe wheezing, whistling, or "noises in my chest when I breathe." Many children will not complain at all. Their parents may notice their child is not keeping up with the other kids at play. Some parents may actually be aware that the child's thorax is hyper-inflated. The manifestations of asthma are protean.

Signs of asthma, especially in the hospital setting, include the expected "wheezing." The wheezing should be *polyphonic* with different pitches or frequencies, some higher, some lower. A *monophonic* pitch usually points to a single obstructed bronchus, which is often due to a cancer. The wheezing in the asthmatic is both inspiratory and expiratory. Other signs of asthma include tachypnea, hyperinflation of the thorax, increased resonance on percussion and decreased breath sounds with severe expiratory slowing. Some patients, especially those who are allergic to aspirin and non-steroidal anti-inflammatory agents may have nasal polyps.

In the office setting, the patient's examination may be normal. If that is the case, the physician must look for symptoms and signs of atopy or allergy such as the typical rash of eczema, a patchy reddish and itchy rash, or signs of allergic rhinitis, a subtle darkening about the eyes (the "allergic shiner"), a runny nose, and a pale, swollen nasal mucosa. Are there Kleenex tissues in her purse or his pocket?

If asthma is suspected, the patient needs to be quizzed about triggers. Did he or she just take aspirin, eat at a restaurant that has a salad bar (some restaurants use Metasulfites to make the salad look good), or play with a neighbor's cat? Does the asthma always occur on the same day of the week? Can the patient identify a potential cause? Some patients are aware of triggers but don't want to admit it. Who wants to give up a cat if they have children who love it?

In the hospital setting when the patient is actively wheezing, the diagnosis can be made by just giving the patient a B adrenergic agent such as albuterol. Does the wheezing improve, and the patient feels better? If so, it is highly likely the patient has asthma. When the patient is in the office and is symptom-free without any signs of asthma, it is more difficult to make a diagnosis of asthma. In that case pulmonary function testing should be done. The typical findings of asthma include:

1. Reduced forced vital capacity (FVC)
2. Reduced forced expiratory volume in one second (FEV1)
3. Markedly reduced FEV1/FVC ratio (less than 70%) due to obstruction of the airways
4. Increased total lung capacity (TLC), due to air trapping
5. Increased residual volume (RV), again due to air trapping
6. Markedly increased RV/TLC ratio
7. Increased FRC due to air trapping. The patient can't exhale the air fully with each breath.
8. Diffusion is normal.

The consequence of the pulmonary function changes is a marked increase in the work of breathing. A greater FRC moves the patient up the pressure/volume or compliance curve so that more pressure or work is needed for a given change in volume.

If the patient has abnormal pulmonary function testing, then a B adrenergic agent is given. If there is a greater than 12% increase in the FEV1 or FVC, the diagnosis is established. If the pulmonary function testing is normal, the patient should have a methacholine challenge test.

Methacholine is an analog of acetyl choline, which is the chemical released by the parasympathetic nervous system. Both methacholine and acetyl choline cause bronchoconstriction by stimulating the production of cyclic GMP (Guanosine mono phosphate). Graduated doses of methacholine are inhaled and the dose which causes a 20% drop in the FEV1 is reported. The test is 95% accurate and 95% specific. Only a recent viral infection or active allergic rhinitis will cause a false positive test.

Often a chest radiograph is done but this test is no longer considered mandatory especially in children in the emergency room. It should only be done when pneumonia is suspected. In adults it should be done initially in the diagnostic workup to exclude other causes of the symptoms such as congestive heart failure, pneumonia, or a cancer.

The sputum should be examined in the acute setting. It should be gram-stained and cultured. The sputum may show Charcot-Leyden crystals which are crystals composed of an eosinophilic protein or Curschmann's spirals which are casts of the small airways and the ducts of the mucous glands. A gram stain and culture of the sputum is needed if a bacterial infection is suspected.

A complete blood count (CBC) may show an increase in neutrophils if there is an infection and an increase in eosinophils, sometimes quite profound, if there is allergy.

Another useful tool is to measure the nitric oxide in the exhaled air, (FeNO or exhaled fraction of nitric oxide). Nitric oxide is produced by the inflamed bronchial tissues. There are many causes of false positive tests including allergic rhinitis so care must be used in evaluating the test results. But the FeNO can help differentiate the H2HI where it is increased from the H2LO where it is normal.

After asthma is diagnosed, its severity should be estimated as this will aid in deciding on the appropriate treatment.

Intermittent asthma is asthma that occurs no more than twice a week, with night-time symptoms no more than twice a month and with an FEV1 greater than 80%. The patient has no limitation of normal activity.

Mild persistent asthma is asthma that has symptoms less than once a day. Night-time symptoms occur about once a week or less. The FEV1 is still more than 80% of predicted and there is only minimal limitation of normal activity.

Moderate persistent asthma is characterized by daily symptoms. Night-time symptoms occur more than once a week. The FEV1 is between 60% and 80% of predicted. There is definite limitation of normal activity.

Severe persistent asthma has continual symptoms which are both daytime and night-time. The FEV1 is less than 60% of predicted. Normal activity is severely impaired. The newest guidelines add the patient should be having asthma even on oral steroids!

While the treatment of asthma is directed at both the bronchospasm and the inflammation, the primary target is inflammation. Because of this, new guidelines for the treatment of asthma have been developed which involve the use of low dose inhaled steroids combined with a B adrenergic agent with even mild intermittent asthma. The guidelines are known as the GINA (Global Strategy for Asthma Management and Prevention) Guidelines and were updated in 2023.

The goals of therapy as outlined by GINA include both symptom control and risk reduction and are as follows:

1. Few asthma symptoms
2. No sleep disturbance
3. No exercise limitation
4. Maintain normal lung function
5. Prevent flare-ups (exacerbations)
6. Prevent asthma deaths
7. Minimize medication side-effects
8. Avoid oral corticosteroids

For intermittent asthma, a long-acting-B adrenergic agent (formoterol) in combination with an inhaled corticosteroid (ICS) is used only as needed. For mild persistent asthma, twice daily low dose ICS-formoterol is used. If this proves inadequate then a moderate dose of ICS-formoterol is used. If the patient has severe persistent asthma, a long-acting-muscarinic agent should be added along with high dose ICS-Formoterol. The patient should be phenotyped and consideration given to the anti-inflammatory antibodies such as anti-IgE, anti-L 4, anti-IL 5, and anti-IL 13 as well as anti-TSLP. Oral corticosteroids is a last resort. The low dose ICS-formoterol combination is always used as a reliever.

The agents used to treat bronchospasm include the B-adrenergic agents, the muscarinic agents, and the theophyllines.

Bronchial tone is affected by both components of the autonomic nervous systems. Stimulation of the adrenergic nervous system causes release of adrenaline or epinephrine which increases the enzyme adenyl cyclase which converts ATP (adenosine triphosphate) into cyclic AMP which then causes bronchodilation. B adrenergic agents mimic the effects of the adrenergic nervous system. Some of the drugs can be given orally, some by inhalation, and some by the intravenous route. Some are short acting, and some are long acting. The list of medications is exceptionally large and includes albuterol, salmeterol, and formoterol. Side effects of these drugs include tachycardia and nervousness. Occasionally there may be a severe cardiac arrhythmia, even ventricular tachycardia.

The Theophyllines also act to increase cyclic AMP. They do this by blocking the enzyme phosphodiesterase which breaks down cyclic AMP into AMP. Blocking the breakdown of cyclic AMP causes bronchodilation. In the past, theophyllines were a mainstay of the treatment of asthma but because of their serious side effects, including cardiac arrhythmias and seizures, they are used much less frequently today. They can be given both orally and intravenously. Of interest, tea, and coffee both contain analogues of the Theophyllines and are potent bronchodilators in their own right.

The parasympathetic nervous system releases acetyl choline which stimulates the production of cyclic GMP from guanosine triphosphate (GTP). Cyclic GMP causes bronchoconstriction. Thus, the anticholinergic or anti-muscarinic agents block acetyl choline from converting GTP into cyclic GMP and by doing so cause bronchodilation. Ipratropium is a short acting anticholinergic and Tiotropium is a long-acting agent. Both are given by inhalation. The main side effects of these drugs in drying of secretions which can, of course, make the mucous thicker and worsen asthma. They should be used carefully in the patient with acute asthma and copious secretions. If the chemicals get into the eye, they can dilate the pupil.

The anti-inflammatory agents include steroids and non-specific anti-leukotriene agents. Steroids are certainly the most effective agents. They suppress bronchial inflammation, but their mechanism of action is unknown. They can be given intravenously in a patient having a severe asthma exacerbation, orally in an outpatient who is having a moderate to severe acute attack, and by inhalation in patients with persistent asthma. Long term oral steroids should be avoided as they cause cataracts, osteoporosis, and hypokalemia. On the other hand, hand-held inhaled steroids are often used continuously. The main side effect is thrush, which is an oral infection with Candida albicans, characterized by white shiny patches on the tongue and walls of the throat.

Non-specific anti-leukotrienes include Singular. The drug modifies the leukotriene pathway and, while mildly effective for allergic rhinitis, is of little value in the treatment of asthma. There is some evidence that Singular can precipitate or worsen depression.

Recently a new class of medication has been introduced. They monoclonal antibodies and can be recognized by the presence of "mab" at the end of their generic name. At the present time there are five main targets of these antibodies. The first, omalizumab, is directed at IgE. It is given every 2-4 weeks subcutaneously. The agent binds free IgE preventing it from binding to the receptor on the mast cell. The agent also down-regulates the mast cell receptor. The drug is effective and reduces the risk of an asthma exacerbation by 38%. Both symptoms and the need for rescue medications fell by more than half in two years. Patients with severe allergic asthma, often with the highest eosinophil count, appear to get the most benefits from the drug.

IL-5 is important in the production, maturation, and activation of eosinophils. In the last 2 or 3 years, three antibodies have been released which are active against IL-5: mepolizumab, Reslizumab, and Benralizumab. The latter agent works by blocking the receptor site for IL-5. All three drugs reduce exacerbations by 50%.

Dupilumab has recently been released. It is directed at both IL-4 and IL-13. It binds to a subunit of the IL-4 receptor and inhibits IL-4 and Il-13. The agent has just been released under the trade name Dupixent. It is to be used in patients with moderate to severe asthma over the age of 12 who have either an eosinophilic phenotype or corticosteroid dependent asthma. It also reduces the risk of exacerbations by 50%.

A new antibody has just been developed that is directed at the Alarmin *TSLP*. It is called Tezepelumab and was released in 2022. It is the first antibody to be directed at the Alarmins and also reduces asthmatic exacerbations by about 50%.

The antibodies are given intravenously and are quite expensive. The main complication with all of the antibodies is a severe anaphylactic reaction. In addition, some patients can develop serious systemic eosinophilia associated with a vasculitis or inflammation of the lining of blood vessels. Because the antibodies suppress the immune response, the use of live vaccines must be avoided in patients taking these agents. Killed vaccines can be used and are effective. In addition, the patient should be checked for tuberculosis and fungal diseases such as histoplasmosis before starting therapy as these diseases may become reactivated.

Bronchial thermoplasty is a recent addition to the anti-asthma regimen. It involves threading a radiofrequency catheter through a bronchoscope which can heat the airway. The radiofrequency waves decrease the amount of airway smooth muscle. In a controlled study, the rates of severe exacerbations, emergency visits, and days missed from work or school was significantly reduced in patients getting the bronchial thermoplasty. There was no effect on lung function itself. Thermoplasty is best used in non-allergic asthmatics.

Atypical phenotypes of asthma include aspirin induced or exacerbated respiratory disease and allergic bronchopulmonary aspergillosis (ABPA).

Aspirin Induced Asthma

The first reported case of aspirin causing an exacerbation of asthma appeared in 1902. In 1968 Max Samter described *Samter's triad* which consists of aspirin sensitivity, nasal polyps, and asthma. Arachidonic acid can be converted to either the prostaglandins, which are for the most part bronchodilators by the enzyme cyclooxygenase, or into the leukotrienes (LTC4, LTD4, and LTE4), which are for the most part bronchoconstrictors by the enzyme 5-lipoxygenase. The non-steroidal anti-inflammatory agents all work by blocking the cyclooxygenase reaction, preventing the conversion of arachidonic acid to the prostaglandins, and increasing the production of leukotrienes causing bronchoconstriction. This reaction is not due to allergy nor is it IgE mediated. This condition is actually fairly common. 7% of asthmatics in general and 14% of severe asthmatics are sensitive to aspirin.

Generally, aspirin allergy begins in adults who first develop a moderately severe, refractory rhinitis with nasal polyps. Then over time the asthma develops. An asthma attack can occur anywhere from 30 minutes to 3 hours after ingesting the nonsteroidal agent. A few patients develop urticarial (hives) or even angioedema. Some patients become sensitive to alcohol as well. In these patients, alcohol will cause either rhinitis or an asthma exacerbation.

The diagnosis is made by giving the patient aspirin in a very controlled environment by doctors who are experts in this area.

These patients do not do as well with conventional therapy although leukotriene therapy with Singular or Montelukast is often added to the regimen. **Aspirin desensitization is effective but once accomplished the patient must always take a full-strength aspirin twice daily**. If the patient stops the aspirin for more than three days, the desensitization must be repeated.

Allergic Bronchopulmonary Aspergillosis (ABPA)

The fungus Aspergillus can cause three distinct syndromes. It can cause a virulent pneumonia which is usually fatal, and which is most often seen in immunocompromised patients such as patients with AIDS. It can form a "fungus ball" and fill a bulla in a patient with emphysema sometimes causing massive hemoptysis. Or it can colonize the bronchial epithelium and cause an allergic reaction leading to asthma, bronchiectasis, and pneumonia. This latter syndrome is known as allergic bronchopulmonary aspergillosis.

ABPA occurs in about 1 in 50 to 1 in 100 patients with asthma. It also occurs in about 5 to 10% of patients with cystic fibrosis. Pathologically the fungal hyphae fill the lumen of bronchial tubes. The fungus does not invade the pulmonary tissue itself. The disease occurs because of the allergic reaction to the fungus. There is a marked increase in IgE and eosinophils due to activation of the Th2 inflammatory pathway.

Patients with ABPA present with the typical symptoms of asthma associated with fever, weakness, and the production of an extremely thick brown mucous which is often described as "so thick you could chew it." Physical signs include those of both asthma and pneumonia.

The laboratory findings are most helpful. There is a marked increase in eosinophils, a remarkably high IgE (>1000 IU/ml), and both IgE and IgG antibodies to the fungus. The sputum may grow Aspergillus fumigatus and the fungal hyphae can be seen on a smear of the sputum.

The chest x-ray and high-resolution CAT scan of the chest often shows signs of bronchiectasis as well as acute pneumonia including "tram lines" and "signet rings."

In order to make the diagnosis the patient must have either asthma or cystic fibrosis and have a positive skin test for aspergillus and an elevated serum IgE in the extremely high range. The patient must have pulmonary findings on the chest radiograph consistent with ABPA, antibodies to the fungus, and a high eosinophil count.

The treatment of ABPA is with oral or intravenous steroids. Most often, the patient will, in fact, require lifetime therapy with oral steroids. Inhaled steroids are generally not effective. If the patient can't be weaned from oral steroids, then an antifungal agent such as Itraconazole can be tried.

Obesity

The primary inflammatory pathway of asthma is via the T-helper 2 lymphocyte. However, recent studies have shown that obesity causes asthma via the T-helper 1 lymphocyte pathway instead. Fat cells are highly inflammatory and the inflammation results in sleep apnea, atherosclerosis, coronary artery disease and strokes. It appears that asthma in an obese patient is neutrophil mediated as opposed to eosinophil mediated in allergic asthma. It also is more likely to occur in women than in men.

The best therapy for asthma related to obesity is to lose weight which will decrease the inflammation. In a study of obese nurses with asthma, as little as a 10 lb. weight loss significantly improved asthma in a substantial number of patients. Other treatments that should be considered are the use of inhaled Tiotropium and continuous Azithromycin orally (500 mg three times a week) though both treatments are still controversial.

Suggestions for minor papers

1. Compare the pulmonary function test results of all the obstructive diseases.
2. What does the eosinophil do?
3. What do the mast cells do and where do they come from?
4. What does cortisone do? How long has it been used to treat asthma?
5. Outline a treatment plan for a patient with asthma.
6. What is an "asthma action plan?"
7. How does obesity cause asthma?
8. Describe the GINA guidelines. How do they differ from the older guidelines?

Three

Pneumonia

The word "pneumonia" comes from the Greek word "Pneumo" which means "air." Pneumonia is a shortened version of the word "pneumonitis" with means literally "inflammation of the air." There are many completely different types of pneumonia or pneumonitides (the plural of pneumonitis), everything from "walking pneumonia" to the pneumonia caused by medications such as Methotrexate to the pneumonia associated with immune complex diseases such as Rheumatoid Arthritis.

There are a few things all these pneumonitides have in common. They all involve the parenchyma of the lung as opposed to the airway. They are all characterized by inflammation of the alveoli and its supporting structure. For that reason, they are all restrictive diseases. The total lung capacity (TLC), vital capacity (VC) and residual volumes (RV) are all reduced. The flow rates, such as the forced expiratory volume in one second (FEV1), may also be reduced but the ratio between the FEV1 and FVC is always normal, or it may even be increased.

For convenience we divide the "pneumonitides" into two large groups: those associated with infection and those not associated with infection. The former includes pneumonias due to bacteria, viruses, fungi, rickettsia, and mycobacterium. The latter group includes "pneumonitides" due to a vascular, granulomatous, or an inflammatory process.

This seminar will discuss the infectious causes of pneumonia. Important points include, firstly, the need to determine the type of organism causing the pneumonia. Is it a bacterium, a virus, a type of tuberculosis, or a fungus such as histoplasmosis or coccidiomycosis? Secondly, if it is a bacterial or viral pneumonia, where did the patient get sick? Did he or she get sick outside the hospital setting? Or did he become ill after being in hospital for more than 48 hours, on dialysis, been on antibiotics in the last 90 days, or is living in a nursing home? Thirdly, is the presentation of the pneumonia acute with shaking chills, cough with phlegm, fever and perhaps pleurisy? Or does it have a more indolent onset presenting instead with weakness, fatigue, a mild cough with clear or scanty phlegm and perhaps even shortness of breath?

Peter A. Petroff, MD

Case Presentations

1

Michael is a 49-year-old electrical engineer who has been on a fishing excursion with his friends for the last week. Their typical day is predictable. They arise at 4 AM, pack their supplies and then board their little boats. They begin fishing at about five and fish until mid-morning. Then they return to the campsite, and have lunch, usually with a few beers. They head back to their boats about 4 PM and fish to seven or eight. Then they have supper, which always involves some alcohol.

The day before Michael came to the hospital, he developed the acute onset of a cough which was productive of rusty colored phlegm. That night he began having shaking chill and a fever. The following morning his friends took him to the emergency room.

In the emergency room, the physician noted that Michael had no history of lung or heart disease. He was not taking any medications. He smoked about a half pack of cigarettes a day and smoked "pot" on occasion. Michael described his drinking as moderate, but the doctor noted he drank two to four drinks of varying types of alcohol almost every day. Michael has been an electrical engineer since he graduated college and works for a major corporation. His family history was positive for diabetes and heart disease.

On examination, Michael appeared short of breath, and he had a temperature of 102 degrees F. His lips were slightly cyanotic. His breathing was rapid and shallow. The doctor noted fine inspiratory crackles over the right lower lobe. As the doctor examined the area where he heard the crackles, Michael said, "That's where it hurts. It hurts when I take a breath…right there" as he pointed at the right side of his chest.

The doctor ordered a chest radiograph, blood count (CBC) and because of the cyanosis and dyspnea arterial blood gases.

The chest radiograph showed a right lower lobe pneumonia but was otherwise unremarkable. The blood count showed a white count of 18,000 with 75% neutrophils and 8% band neutrophils. The blood gases showed a pO2 of 64, a pCO2 of 35, a pH or 7.48 and an HCO3 of 24.

After getting the laboratory report, the doctor admitted Michael to the hospital. He began him on oxygen at two liters per nasal cannula, intravenous fluids, and Levaquin by IV. Levaquin is a fluoroquinolone antibiotic. He also ordered a blood culture, sputum culture and a procalcitonin level.

By the late afternoon, Michael became still more short of breath and confused. When the doctor returned, Michael was agitated and disorientated. He was more cyanotic. He also appeared to be in pain, frequently grabbing for his right side. The doctor immediately ordered another set of ABGs and transferred Michael to the ICU.

The ABGs showed a pO2 of 43, a pCO2 of 54, a pH of 7.32 and a HCO3 of 24.

In the ICU, the doctor changed the O2 to a 100% non-rebreathing mask and gave the patient Versed, a mild sedation intravenously. Because Michael's color did not improve, the doctor intubated him and placed him on a ventilator. He was placed on an assist control of 10 with 100% oxygen and a tidal volume of 500 ccs. (100 kg X 5 cc/kg).

Michael relaxed almost immediately, and his color improved. After a few minutes, a chest radiograph was done which showed the endotracheal tube in good position. The pneumonia was unchanged. Blood gases showed a pO2 of 350 and the 100% oxygen was decreased to 40%.

Over the next three days, Michael's condition improved. The blood and sputum cultures both showed Streptococcus pneumoniae. The procalcitonin was initially quite high but by the third day was nearly normal. He was extubated on the fourth day and was able to go home after just a week in the hospital. He was seen in the clinic in one month. At that time, the chest radiograph was nearly normal.

2.

David is a sixty-year-old male. He states he has been out of work "as long as I can remember." He lives out of a grocery cart on the south side of the city. He drinks and smokes, "whatever I can get my hands on." He is pleasant, affable, and despite his circumstances, actually quite happy. He was brought to the ER by the police who picked him up off the streets the night before. It was going to be a very cold night and the police wanted to get anyone they could some shelter. The police officer noted that David had a severe cough productive of large amounts of phlegm and some of the phlegm was bloody.

In the ER, David had a low-grade temperature (100.8 degrees F) and an obvious productive cough. A nurse, after hearing the cough and seeing David, put him in a private room in the ER. She then told the rest of the staff to "mask and glove up" when they entered the room and make sure they wash their hands after taking off their gloves.

The doctor noted that David did not take any medications. He had a history of minor surgery in the past but was unsure what kind of surgery it was or where it was done. He could not recall being in the hospital. His father died with pneumonia when he was a child. David was raised in an orphanage. The patient did not know what a PPD was much less whether he had ever had one.

The doctor examined David. He noted that the patient was thin, almost wasted. He did not appear pale or cyanotic. He used his accessory muscles to breathe. His lungs showed diffuse coarse crackles throughout all lung fields which cleared with a deep cough which was productive of blood-tinged greenish phlegm.

The doctor ordered a chest radiograph, blood gases, a blood count, a sputum culture, and a sputum for Tuberculosis (sputum for AFB or acid-fast bacilli).

The chest radiograph showed fibro-calcific changes in the right upper lobe with a calcified nodule in the mid-left lung field. The complete blood count showed a normal white count and a mild anemia. The blood gases were essentially normal. The cultures were still pending.

After reviewing the chest radiograph, the physician admitted David to the hospital in an isolation room. He also did a PPD. He began David on four antibiotics: Isoniazid, Rifampin, Ethambutol, and Pyrazinamide as well as Vitamin B6.

By the second day after admission, the PPD was positive (over 15 mm) and the sputum stain showed acid fast bacilli consistent with tuberculosis. The medications were continued while plans were made for David's post hospital care. He would have to take antibiotics for several months and because of his lifestyle, these would have to be monitored closely. The health department was called in to help. The caseworker spoke with David at length about his friends hoping to be able to find any close contacts who should also be tested for TBC.

David followed the instructions surprisingly well and took his medications regularly under supervision. He completed all nine months of therapy. His cough completely disappeared.

3.

Ellen G. is a twenty-two-year-old gravida 1, para 0. She is eight months pregnant. She is brought to the emergency room by her husband because of fever, cough, and shortness of breath. Because of her shortness of breath and some degree of confusion he gives most of the history. He states that the pregnancy has been uneventful. She has seen the doctor every month and taken her prenatal vitamins regularly. They are the only medications she is taking. Her vital signs including her blood pressure have been normal. She didn't even have morning sickness. The fetus is a boy and appears on ultrasound to be totally normal. Neither he nor his wife have any history of cystic fibrosis or other genetic diseases. She does not smoke or drink or use recreational drugs.

She works as a nurse at a hospital. She remembers taking care of a patient with pneumonia the week before. Two days ago, she developed a sore throat, headache, and irritating cough. She stayed home from work because of it. Yesterday she developed a fever and began getting a little short of breath. This morning, she awakened with severe shortness of breath and fever. There was some nausea as well. As soon as he saw his wife, her husband bundled her up and drove her to the hospital.

Her past history is totally unremarkable. She has no history of any surgery or medical illnesses. She has no history of heart disease or lung disease. Both her parents are living and well. She has worked as a nurse for the last year after graduating from college. Her husband said that she did get a flu shot.

Her physical examination reveals her to be confused, mildly agitated, and diaphoretic. Her lips and fingertips are cyanotic. Her blood pressure is 96/74, her pulse is 108 and her oxygen saturation is 84% on room air. Her height and weight could not be done.

The doctor orders a CBC, chemistry profile, screening test for influenza, a chest radiograph and arterial blood gases. He begins her on a high flow nasal cannula.

The chest radiograph shows a right lower lobe pneumonia, but the radiologist is concerned that the pneumonia may be bilateral. There are also some interstitial changes in the left lung though they were mild. The CBC showed a white cell count of only 2500 (N = 5000-10000), the hemoglobin and platelet count were normal. There are 25% band cells on the differential. The paO2 is 94 on oxygen; the paCO2 is 34; the pH is 7.45. The screening test for influenza (rapid influenza antigen test) is negative. The chemistry panel is normal including the sugar and renal function tests (BUN and Creatinine).

The doctor admits her to the ICU, inserts a feeding tube, begins her on Oseltamivir (Tamiflu: 75 mg bid per nasogastric tube), Zithromycin and Augmentin (both intravenously). He also orders a nucleic acid amplification test (rPT-PCR) for influenza. He continues the oxygen and begins intravenous fluids.

The next morning, she is even more dyspneic. The chest radiograph is worse. There is an interstitial process involving all the lung fields. Her pO2 drops to 64. There are signs of fetal distress on the fetal monitor. The patient is intubated and placed on a ventilator with settings: 90% O2, AC of 12, TV of 400 cc (estimated weight 50 kg) and a PEEP of 5. She is sedated with a Propofol drip.

Her obstetrician is called. He deems the fetus to be viable and says he is available if needed to perform an emergency Cesarean section.

After she is intubated her pO2 increased to 225 and the fiO2 is decreased to 60%. The O2 saturation is still greater than 90. The fetal heart rate returns to a normal range. The patient's blood pressure is 110/84 with a pulse of 92.

Later in the day, the PCR test for influenza shows that Ellen has a H1N1 influenza. The white blood count increases to 10,500 and there are fewer bands. The Tamiflu is continued as were the antibiotics.

Over the next two days, Ellen improves. The oxygen was tapered to 40%. The course of antiviral medication is stopped on the fifth day.

On the sixth hospital day she is extubated. She is discharged home two days later. The following month she has an uncomplicated delivery of a 7-pound, 10-ounce boy.

4. (a pediatric case study)

David is a usually quite healthy 3-month-old infant who was brought to the emergency room by his mother with a runny nose (rhinorrhea) and shortness of breath, as shown by faster respiratory rate. For the last three days, David has not been drinking well, and his mom tells the doctor he has not wet his diaper in the last eight hours. He has not had any gastrointestinal symptoms such as vomiting or diarrhea.

Both David's parents work, and David is cared for during the day by a daycare center. The mother tells the doctor that several of the other children at the care center have been ill in the last two weeks, but none have been hospitalized.

David has not had a cough, but his mom says he has had some "rattling" in his chest.

The mom says that David is her first child. He was the product of a normal pregnancy and delivery. He weighed 7 lbs. at birth, his height was at the 60th percentile, and his Apgar score was normal. He normally consumes 4-5 ounces of breast milk or formula every four hours and produces 8-10 dirty diapers a day.

Neither of the parents smoke. Smoking is not allowed at the daycare center. Neither parent has a history of lung disease including asthma. The mother did not get an RSV vaccine during the pregnancy. "I don't believe in vaccines."

David has a temperature of 101 F. His B/P is 82/50, his respiratory rate is 52, and his pulse is 148. His O2 saturation is 88% on room air. Although he is drowsy, he appears dyspneic in mild to moderate respiratory distress. He has a runny nose, nasal flaring, and his conjunctiva is injected. There are coarse breath sounds with bilateral wheezing, both inspiratory and expiratory. There are intercostal retractions. The examination of his abdomen, extremities, and neurological system are normal except for the drowsiness.

The doctor begins David on oxygen and inserts an IV to give him fluids. His oxygen saturation increases to 93%. He also gives David an albuterol treatment. A chest radiograph is done as are blood tests for a CBC, chemistry profile, and testing for influenza, COVID, and RSV. He admits David to the infant ICU with a diagnosis of bronchiolitis most likely due to the respiratory syncytial virus. He is begun on IV fluids, oxygen, Tylenol suppositories for fever, isolation, and cardiopulmonary monitoring. The albuterol is changed to racemic epinephrine. The radiologist said that the chest x-ray is normal.

The next morning, David appears more dyspneic and his O2 saturation has fallen to 88%. Arterial blood gases showed a PaO2 of 54, a PaCO2 of 54 and a pH of 7.24. He was placed on nasal continuous positive airway pressure (CPAP) with a pressure of 5 cm. The O2 saturation increased to 90% and the CPAP was increased to 10 cm. He was changed from oxygen to heliox or a helium-oxygen gas mixture. In addition, treatments with 5% hypertonic saline was added.

Over the next several days, David got better, and by the fifth day he was using a nasal cannula. Three days later he was discharged.

Seminars in Respiratory Disease

Background for the Presentation

These four cases illustrate different aspects of the disease "pneumonia." In the first case we have a "typical" pneumonia, community acquired, due Streptococcus pneumoniae. In the second case we have a patient with a more indolent type of pneumonia caused by Mycobacterium Tuberculosis. The third patient had pneumonia and respiratory failure due to the influenza virus while the last patient was an infant with a respiratory syncytial virus infection.

IMPORTANT POINTS:

1. Bacterial pneumonia usually results from either aspiration of bacteria or from blood-borne bacteria.
2. The airways of the lungs are not sterile. Our lungs have a **microbiome**.
3. Pneumonia is generally classified by the organism that causes the disease but often the organism is not known. Because of that, we must distinguish between pneumonia that is acquired in the community and pneumonia acquired in a hospital, nursing home or in a patient recently on antibiotics or who is on dialysis.
4. We also classify pneumonia by its presentation. Is it a "typical" pneumonia which is characterized by an acute onset of a high fever, shaking chills, a cough with phlegm and chest pain? Or is it "atypical" with a gradual onset over a few days, profound weakness and malaise, slight cough with perhaps clear or scanty phlegm, and shortness of breath? The treatment of pneumonia depends upon knowing where the pneumonia occurred as well as the identity of the organism causing the disease. In most cases, the treatment will also depend upon the sensitivity of the organism to different antibiotics.
5. The chest radiograph will give us the most amount of information. It will tell us whether there is pneumonia, whether it is localized or diffuse, and whether it appears more chronic than acute. It will tell us if there is an associated disease process such as congestive heart failure, COPD, or cancer.
6. The screening test for influenza is only about 50% sensitive. The PCR test is much more accurate, but it takes several hours to days to get the results.
7. Doxycycline, Fluoroquinolones, and Biaxin should be avoided in the pregnant patient because of the risk of bone disease in the fetus.
8. Influenza can cause pneumonia by itself although many patients were believed to have died of a superimposed bacterial pneumonia during the 1918 influenza pandemic. This was likely not true. The patients died of pneumonia due to the virus.
9. H1N1 influenza affected mainly infants, pregnant women, and patients who were immunocompromised.
10. The Coronavirus is the most common cause of a "cold," but in the last twenty years it has caused three pandemics, SARS 1, MERS, and, most recently, Covid 19. The virus mutates very frequently. That is why a woman with a school age child can have a cold nearly every month.

Discussion

As recently as twenty years ago, the trachea and large airways were thought to be sterile but they, in fact, have their own **biome** or collection of bacteria. The biome occurs because we frequently (several times a day, especially at night) aspirate small amounts of bacteria from our mouths (called immigration) and then clear the bacteria (called removal) by either the bactericidal chemicals present in the mucous lining of the airways or by the mucociliary ladder propelling the mucous to the larynx where we cough it out. It is only when we become more susceptible to infection, perhaps because of the effects of aging or the lack of immunity caused by medication or disease, that pneumonia occurs.

If the invading organism is able to penetrate to the smallest airways and the alveoli, it sets off an intense inflammatory reaction. The mast cells proliferate and attack the foreign body. These cells then release chemicals called **cytokines** which enter the bloodstream and signal neutrophils and lymphocytes to come to the site of the invasion. The "helper" or "T4" lymphocytes determine the antigenic nature of the surface of the invading organism and signal the plasma cells to create antibodies against the antigens. The antibodies then coat the surface of the invader allowing the neutrophils to engulf and destroy the organism by releasing enzymes called "proteinases." Fluid is drawn along with the cellular infiltrate and the involved lung becomes red and heavy, a condition called "red hepatization" or "consolidation" because the lung has the weight and feel of the liver. If the patient survives, the lung will gradually, at least in most types of pneumonia, return to normal.

There are two ways of classifying pneumonia. Is it community acquired, or hospital acquired? Is it a typical pneumonia or an atypical pneumonia?

Community acquired pneumonia is seen in otherwise healthy individuals. The patients are not in the hospital or, if in the hospital, have been there for less than 48 hours before developing signs and symptoms of pneumonia. They have not been on antibiotics in the last 3 months. They are not on dialysis. They are not residing in a nursing home. There are several common bacterial and viral culprits which can cause community acquired pneumonia:

1. Streptococcus pneumoniae
2. Hemophilus influenzae
3. Mycoplasma pneumoniae
4. Legionella pneumophilia
5. Chlamydia pneumonia
6. Orthomyxoviridae influenza
7. Respiratory syncytial virus
8. Coronavirus

The first two cause "typical" pneumonias; the last six cause "atypical" pneumonias. A typical pneumonia is characterized by the abrupt onset of fever, chills (usually described as "shaking"), cough with phlegm (usually purulent and sometimes bloody) and chest pain or pleurisy. The pain is localized over the area of the pneumonia. The chest x-ray shows a focal lesion either *"lobar"* with consolidation over an entire lobe of the lung, or *"bronchial"* with multiple areas of consolidation. An "atypical" pneumonia is characterized by a much slower onset and the main symptom is malaise which can often be profound. The patient may have a low-grade temperature and an irritating cough productive of scanty amounts of clear phlegm. He or she may feel chilly but does not have shaking chills. He or she may have chest pain, but the pain is usually more generalized and is due to muscle pain from the irritating, incessant cough. The chest radiograph shows a diffuse infiltrate consistent with the acute respiratory distress syndrome (ARDS).

Certainly, **pneumococcal pneumonia** is the most common cause of community acquired pneumonia. It causes a typical pneumonia. It is caused by Streptococcus pneumoniae or the "diplococcus." The term "Streptococcus" is the name of the genus to which the organism belongs. The term "pneumoniae" is the "species." The genus is always capitalized; the species is not. Under the microscope the organism appears to be two spheres attached to each other. They are always found inside infected cells. Hence, they were at one time known as "intracellular diplococci."

The cocci or round bacteria, as opposed to the bacilli or rod-like bacteria, consist of two common genera: Streptococcus and Staphylococcus. The Streptococci occur either as diplococci or in chains such as in "Beta Strep" which causes "Strep Throat." The Staphylococci occur in bunches of cocci. I call them the "grapes of wrath." All cocci have thick cell walls and stain blue with the Gram stain; at one time, all were sensitive to penicillin. At the present time some of the Staphylococci in the species "aureus" are resistant to penicillin and are called "Methicillin Resistant Staph aureus" or MRSA. In addition, in the United States, even St. pneumoniae is often resistant to the macrolides such as Zithromycin.

Hemophilus influenzae is an organism whose shape is in between the sphere-like cocci and the rod-like bacilli. Hence it is called a coccobacillus. When it was first discovered in 1892, it was thought to be the cause of Influenza or the flu and therefore given its name. In fact, it wasn't until the 1930's when the flu was found to be due to a virus. Hemophilus influenzae type b can survive well with or without oxygen and the organism is commonly found living harmlessly in the mouth. Children, the elderly and the immunologically impaired can become ill due to the bacterium. It normally presents as a typical pneumonia, but with less fever and cough.

Mycoplasma pneumoniae is the most important cause of "atypical pneumonia" in young adults. In fact, it accounts for 40% of all community acquired pneumonia. The patient presents with a low-grade fever, headache, sore throat, irritating cough or a cough with scanty phlegm, and generalized malaise. Often the illness lasts for several weeks. It seems to be so mild it is frequently called walking pneumonia." It usually affects college-age students. The organism is so small that it cannot be seen under a light microscope. It has no cell wall. At one time it was thought to be a virus. It has limited ability to reproduce on its own and thus is a parasite depending upon the host cells for reproduction. It fuses with the host cell, invades the cell, and then lives inside the cell using the metabolism of the host to reproduce. Because it is able to survive inside the cell, it evades the common defenses of the body and can survive in the cell for weeks to months.

Legionnaire's disease is caused by **Legionella pneumophilia**. Legionnaire's disease (LD) was first recognized in 1976 during an outbreak of **a severe pneumonia occurring** at an American Legion convention in Philadelphia. The pneumonia did not respond to conventional antibiotics and the fatality rate was quite high. The organism was later found to be a bacillus which stained red on the Gram stain (Gram-negative). Legionnaire's disease affects mainly the elderly. It accounts for up to 15% of community acquired pneumonias that result in hospitalization. Of particular note, the organism can survive and be transmitted in air conditioning systems, cooling towers, showers, and even respiratory therapy equipment. Because of that it has caused very severe outbreaks of pneumonia in hospitals. Like the Mycoplasma, the organism survives intracellularly. The alveolar macrophages ingest the organism but cannot kill it. Instead, it uses the host cell as a source for its metabolites. The symptoms resemble those of Mycoplasma, but diarrhea is frequently seen and is a hallmark of the disease.

Chlamydophila pneumoniae is a tiny (about the same size as the Mycoplasma organism), gram-negative bacillus, which like both Legionella and Mycoplasma survives well inside the alveolar macrophages. It has been associated with asthma, lung cancer, and even central nervous system diseases such as multiple sclerosis, although, with the exception of asthma, the association appears to be weak.

Influenza is caused by the organism, Orthomyxoviridae influenza, which has several subspecies, Type A, B, C and D. Type A and B are the most common and Type A is the most common cause of severe "influenza." It is an RNA virus which means that instead of using DNA to reproduce the organism uses the RNA molecule. The influenza type A virus is further classified based on two surface proteins called **hemagglutinin (HA or H)** and **neuraminidase (NA or N)**. The cause of the severe epidemic of 1918 which killed upwards of 60,000,000 people was the H1N1 virus which also caused the epidemic in 2009. The symptoms of the flu vary widely. They range from a sore throat with aches and pains, low grade fever, mild headache and an irritating cough that last a few days to an illness characterized by the abrupt onset of fever, cough and shortness of breath that is fatal within twenty-four hours.

The **Respiratory Syncytial Virus (RSV)** was first identified in 1957. It was found to be the cause of bronchiolitis in children. However, in the 1980's, it was also identified as a cause of pneumonia in adults. It is an Orthopneumovirus. It is similar to the flu in many respects. It most often causes an upper respiratory infection or bronchiolitis in infants but can also cause pneumonia in the elderly. Typical symptoms in the young baby include a runny nose, cough, sneezing, fever, and wheezing. Neither Covid nor influenza cause wheezing. The organism is transmitted by aerosolized droplets or by coming in contact with fomites on hard surfaces on which the organism can survive for days. It enters the body through the eyes, nose, or mouth. Infections peak in winter in the Northern Hemisphere.

Infected cells fuse to each other and to uninfected cells forming syncytia which are giant multinucleated cells, spreading the viral progeny.

Like the common cold due to the coronavirus, immunity is **short-lived**. RSV is actually more severe and more common in adults than the flu. In the elderly, RSV causes 14,000 deaths a year, especially adults with cardiopulmonary disease. 10-31% of infections require ICU admission, 3-17% require mechanical ventilation, and 6-8% die! In a study by Dr. Falsey published in the New England Journal of Medicine, both healthy adults and adults with cardiopulmonary disease were 2.5 times as likely to get RSV as to get the flu and between 4 and 10% of the high-risk patients got RSV yearly. RSV accounts for 11% of pneumonias in adults and 11% of COPD exacerbations. The RSV can be diagnosed with a nasal or pharyngeal swab similar to coronavirus. The test is called the PCR test and is 95% sensitive. If an older individual goes to the ER with a pneumonia, most likely he will get a "Multiplexed influenza, coronavirus, RSV PCR test.

PCR stands for "polymerase chain reaction." The test can detect very tiny amounts of genetic material from an invading organism. The test is done by sampling blood or sputum or obtaining nasal smear. The sample contains the patient's DNA as well as the DNA or RNA from the virus. If the virus is an RNA virus it must first be treated with Reverse Transcriptase, an enzyme which converts RNA into DNA. The sample is then exposed to an enzyme called polymerase which multiplies the amount of DNA present. Within an hour there will be billions of copies of the organism's DNA which can be identified. The test has also been used to detect cancer cells.

RSV bronchiolitis is a cause of childhood asthma. The risk of asthma persists at least to age 7 and is 30% higher than infants who have not had RSV. RSV may also cause bronchiolitis obliterans and thrombocytopenia.

There is no specific treatment at the present time for RSV, but several vaccines are available or will soon be available. Every pregnant woman should get the RSV vaccine unless there is a contraindication because the newborn depends on the mother's antibodies for the first six months of its life. In addition, newborns and the elderly should be vaccinated as well. The vaccine has been shown to decrease severe symptoms by 80% and any symptom by 70%. The vaccine targets the RSV glycoprotein prefusion conformation on the surface of the virus. There is no specific treatment as of yet for RSV.

Treatment is largely providing symptomatic relief, administering antipyretics, IV fluids, oxygen, and appropriate respiratory therapy which may include ventilator care and even ECMO. Droplet and contact isolation precautions should be taken to prevent the spread of the disease.

Inhaled ribavirin can be used in severely ill patients but is only weakly effective.

A case of **Coronavirus pneumonia** is presented in the seminar dealing with ARDS. The Coronavirus is a common RNA virus that most often causes the common cold. Other causes of colds include the Adenovirus which is a DNA virus and the Rhinovirus which is also an RNA virus. However, three types of the coronavirus have appeared in the last twenty years that have caused severe respiratory disease. The first was SARS or **Severe Acute Respiratory Syndrome**. It began in China in 2002-3 likely when a bat transferred the disease to a human via a civet cat, though ferret badgers, domestic cats, and raccoon dogs could also have been infected. It affected 8000 people of which 800 died. Overall, there was a 9% mortality. Most of the cases were in Hong Kong and China but there was at least one case in Toronto and one in Houston. One hospital in Toronto was put on total lockdown to prevent the disease from spreading. Patients, nurses, doctors, respiratory therapists, and other staff were confined to the hospital for more than a week.

The second outbreak of a Coronavirus infection called **Middle Eastern Acute Respiratory Syndrome,** was identified in Saudi Arabia in 2012. The disease even spread to the United States. This disease appears to have originated in bats but was communicated first to camels and then to humans. As of January of 2020, there were 2519 cases with 866 deaths. The illness is rare but still prevalent in the Middle East.

The current Coronavirus infection (**Covid 19**) began in a food market in Wuhan, China likely in bats which spread the disease to civet cats or pangolins and then to humans in early December of 2019. Hence, it is called Covid 19 for Coronavirus disease, 2019. To date it has infected more than 567 million people world-wide and caused more than six million deaths. More than a million Americans have died from the disease and 90 million have been infected as of July 21, 2022.

While the original Covid 19 virus caused the most severe disease, as the virus has mutated it has become less virulent and more contagious. There have been several subspecies, most recently Omicron Ba5 and Ba4. The virus continues to mutate frequently and cause numerous hospitalizations world-wide.

The Covid-19 virus is an RNA virus, which means that it must invade host cells in order to reproduce. Within just a few weeks after the first case appear, on January 8, 2020, the Chinese identified the RNA structure of the virus and published the findings.

The virus is called the coronavirus because the virus particles have club-shaped glycolated-protein spikes that under the electron microscope look like crowns. The virus is spherical and contains a single strand of RNA with 15 genes and 30,000 bases. The influenza virus has only 15,000 bases. The spikes of the virus attach to the ACE-2 (angiotensin converting enzyme-2) receptors located on the surface of cells found in the lung and nose. The virus then invades the cell (a process called endocytosis) releasing its RNA which the host cell replicates generating new viruses which are then released from the cell, free to invade other cells.

Unlike most coronaviruses, the Covid-19 virus does not cause cold-like symptoms. Instead, the symptoms include loss of smell in over 80% of patients (10% of patients with the virus present with only the loss of smell), cough, fever, muscle aches and pains, shortness of breath, nausea, and diarrhea. Surprisingly, the Omicron variant infrequently causes loss of smell and taste. The virus can also cause an inflammation of the heart muscle called myocarditis. The virus can even invade brain tissue and cause neurologic disorders. The virus elicits an immune response but sometimes the immune response can be overwhelming. This is referred to as a "cytokine storm." It is characterized by lymphopenia due to atrophy of the lymphoid tissue, vasculitis (inflammation of the blood vessels), uncontrolled clotting of the blood resulting in gangrene and strokes, and finally multiorgan failure and death. About 30% of patients who survive an acute Covid infection will develop "long covid" which is characterized by prolonged weakness, headache, malaise (often post-exercise), fever, cough, shortness of breath, chest pain, difficulty sleeping, dizziness, depression, confusion, as well as some gastrointestinal symptoms.

The virus is highly contagious. The average person with the disease will spread it to 2.2 others. However, the Omicron variant, an infected person can infect more than 20 people. For contrast, the value for influenza, called the R0 value or "basic reproduction value" is 1.2. For measles it is 12-18 indicating just infective measles is. General, contact, and aerosol precautions are needed to help slow the spread of the disease. The diagnosis is made by obtaining specimens from the nose and posterior pharynx and identifying the organism by either a rapid screen or the PCR test. The rapid screen test results can be back in a few minutes but will miss about 15% of cases.

Treatment at the present time includes Paxlovid which is taken orally for five days if the patient has no more than fever. Recently, a new drug similar to Paxlovid but costing one fourth of the cost of Paxlovid has been developed in China. Simnotrelvir is an oral 3-chymotrypsin–like protease inhibitor that has been found to have in vitro activity against severe acute respiratory syndrome coronavirus 2 (SARS-CoV-2) and potential efficacy in a phase 1B trial.

If, despite treatment with Paxlovid, the patient becomes dyspneic and especially in older patients or patients who are immunocompromised, Nirmatrelvir-ritonavir or Remdesivir have been shown to be effective in moderately severe Covid-19 disease. A cortisone, dexamethasone, has been shown to be helpful in ventilator-dependent patients, reducing the risk of death by 20%. In addition, the plasma of patients that have recovered from the infection has been used to treat severely ill patients as have specific antibodies. More recently, the administration of mesenchymal stromal cells has been shown to improve outcomes in patients with the disorder.[1] Overall, the mortality in the USA is about 4.7%. Compare that to influenza where the mortality is 0.1%. Thus Covid-19 is 47 times more lethal than the flu.

Prevention is the key and involves everyone using a mask, maintaining social distancing as well as intensive testing and contact tracing and quarantining of contacts. In addition, proper hand washing and avoiding contact between your hand and your face are particularly important. Where these measures have been done effectively (China, Korea, New Zealand, Viet Nam, and to a lesser extent Australia, the disease has been controlled. Where it has not, the disease has killed tens of thousands of people. Several vaccines are available some of which are based on mRNA (messenger RNA). At the present time, patients who are immunocompromised or are over 65 should get a total of five doses of the mRNA vaccine (as of September 2023).

It is important to diagnosis the pneumonia as community acquired because all the organisms save the influenza virus, RSV, and Covid can be treated with either a Fluoroquinolone antibiotic such as Levaquin or a macrolide antibiotic such as Zithromycin though the latter agent is not used as often nowadays because of resistance. The most recent recommendations by the American Thoracic Society

---

[1] Chen, Ching-Yi, et al; The Clinical Efficacy and safety of mesenchymal stromal cells for patients with Covid 19; Journal of Infection and Public Health, 15 (202), 896-901

suggest that amoxicillin or amoxicillin-clavulanic, both types of penicillin, are a better choice because of the increased incidence of resistance of the pneumococcus to the macrolides and the many, and often severe, side effects of the Fluoroquinolones. If an atypical organism is suspected then doxycycline, a type of tetracycline could be used. Influenza pneumonia is treated with an antiviral agent such as oseltamivir (Tamiflu) or Zanamivir (Relenza).

Hospital acquired pneumonia is diagnosed in patients who develop pneumonia having been in the hospital for at least 48 hours. It is also seen in patients receiving dialysis, residing in a nursing home, or who have recently taken antibiotics (within 90 days). It also includes patients who are on a ventilator. There are several types of organisms that cause the disease:

1. MRSA or Methicillin Resistant Staph Aureus
2. Pseudomonas aeruginosa
3. Other gram-negative bacilli including Enterobacter
4. Aspiration of gastric contents

The reason to distinguish between hospital acquired pneumonia and community acquired pneumonia is that the treatment is different. Pneumonia in a hospital setting is most often due to highly resistant organisms and must be treated with quite different antibiotics from those used in community acquired pneumonia. MRSA is treated with Vancomycin. Pseudomonas and other gram-negative bacilli are treated with fourth generation penicillins such as Carbenicillin and Ticarcillin as well as cephalosporins including Ceftazidime and Cefepime.

Pseudomonas aeruginosa is a gram-negative bacillus. It is found in our body's warm and moist locations such as our ear canal and the soles of our feet. For the same reason it thrives on medical equipment. It is an opportunistic organism searching out the ideal immunocompromised host. One in ten hospital acquired pneumonias are due to the Pseudomonas. It is also seen ubiquitously in patients with Cystic Fibrosis. It causes a typical pneumonia. The patient infected by Pseudomonas aeruginosa typically has the abrupt onset of fever and cough. The sputum is green and is described as "sweet smelling." The patient who is intubated and on a ventilator usually develops a new fever. The chest x-ray shows a new area of patchy consolidation. The organism is becoming more and more resistant to antibiotics. Culture and antibiotic sensitivity testing must always be done.

Aspiration of gastric contents is quite important, especially in patients who are on ventilators. The consequence of the aspiration depends solely on the pH of the aspirate. If the pH is less than two, there will be a severe chemical burn involving both the large and small airways. The airway inflammation will cause atelectasis and mismatching of ventilation and perfusion. Bacterial contamination is unlikely in the first 48 hours after the aspiration. Treatment is supportive. Prevention is the key. The head of the bed of a ventilated patient must always be elevated at least 30 degrees.

Other organisms which cause pneumonia include the Mycobacteria species and certain fungi:

1. Mycobacterium tuberculosis
2. Mycobacterium avium

3. Coccidioides immitis
4. Histoplasma capsulatum
5. Pneumocystis jiroveci (carinii)

Mycobacterium tuberculosis, the cause of tuberculosis (TBC), is the most common and the most fatal infectious organism in the world. 25% of the world's people are infected with the organism. In 2017 there were more than 10,000,000 active cases of TBC throughout the world and more than 1 and ½ million people died of the disease. Most cases of TBC are found in Asia including China, Indonesia, India, Pakistan, and the Philippines.

The organism is an aerobic rod-like bacterium. Its cell wall is characterized by the presence of mycolic acid which gives it a waxy coat and makes it impervious to the Gram stain. Instead it is stained using an acid-fast stain such as Ziehl-Nielsen stain, or a fluorescent stain such as auramine. Because of its acid-fast staining it is referred to as "acid-fast bacillus" or "AFB." The organism grows very slowly in culture taking up to six weeks to be identified but "nucleic acid-amplification" which uses a positive smear for AFB can identify the organism in just two days.

Mycobacterium tuberculosis only affects human beings. It is spread by air droplets but is highly infectious. Singing is the most efficacious means of spreading the disease.

In the lungs, the organism is deposited in the terminal and respiratory bronchioles. The alveolar macrophages take up the organism but are unable to kill it. The organism multiplies inside the macrophage and then the newly created organisms are released into the tissue and blood. A severe inflammatory response ensues. Macrophages, neutrophils and fibrocytes are attracted to the site of the infection. A chest radiograph taken at this time will show a lobar pneumonia, usually involving the lower or middle lung field. Gradually, over a period of a few weeks, the body develops immunity to the organism and a tumor-like nodular structure called a "granuloma," made up of fibrous tissue, macrophages, and giant cells, is able to isolate the organism. The center of the granuloma is dead tissue which looks like cheese. Hence it is called "caseous necrosis." The patient will now test positive for the tuberculosis antigen although 20% of patients with active Tuberculosis will have a negative test. The skin test is called the PPD (Purified Protein Derivative). A chest x-ray at this stage of the disease will show a pulmonary nodule which will eventually calcify as well as a large hilar lymph node. This is called the Ghon complex. The organism will lie dormant inside the granuloma for years until the patient's immunity level is impaired by age or illness. The organism will then activate and generally cause a pneumonia involving the apical and apical-posterior segments of the upper lobes, but it can also involve the brain, bones, kidneys, or other organ systems.

When the organism first invades the lungs, it also spreads to other tissues such as the meninges, pleura, and bones. Some patients develop meningitis, and some develop pleural effusion and a few have fractures of the spine referred to as Pott's disease.

All medical staff should be tested for the disease by either the PPD or interferon-gamma release assay (IFN-Gamma) which is a blood test that is much more specific than the PPD. In fact, it is more than 95% specific for tuberculosis though it is only about 80% sensitive. Interferon-γ release assays rely on the fact that T-lymphocytes will release IFN-γ when exposed to specific tubercular antigens. If the health care worker has a positive PPD already, then a chest radiograph should be done immediately and annually thereafter. **A positive PPD means the patient has or had tuberculosis.**

BCG or the Bacille-Calmette-Guerin, is a vaccine for tuberculosis. It is given to children in countries where there is a high incidence of TBC such as the Philippines. It is only about 80% effective at preventing an infection. After the injection, the PPD will be positive, but the positivity will wane in less than a decade. If a patient from the Philippines has a positive PPD years after he or she was given the BCG vaccine, be suspicious that the patient actually has or has had active tuberculosis.

The treatment of tuberculosis involves a cocktail of four drugs taken for two to months and then three drugs for an additional seven months but treatment regimens are changing. At the present the patient is started on Isoniazid (INH), Rifampin (RMP), Ethambutol (EMB), and Pyrazinamide (PYZ). In addition, the patient is also given Vitamin B6 to prevent nerve damage from the INH. After two months the EMB is stopped while the other drugs are continued.

Most importantly, every patient with symptoms of cough and phlegm lasting more than a few weeks should at least be considered as having TBC. Isolation in the hospital setting for droplet spread is paramount.

There are several other strains of Mycobacterium including M. avium which causes bronchiectasis (Lady Wyndemere's Syndrome), and M. kansansii which colonizes bullae in patients with emphysema. M. avium can cause a septic infection in patients with AIDS.

Coccidioides immitis is the cause of "Valley Fever," a fungal infection first identified in the central valley of California. It usually causes a very mild flu-like infection lasting just a few days. In certain patients, mainly Blacks and Filipinos, it can cause a fatal systemic infection.

The organism is found in the soil not only in the central valley of California, but in Arizona, New Mexico, southern Texas (as far north as the San Antonio area) and northern Mexico. After a dry spell following a rain, the spores of the fungus are released into the air and are inhaled causing the infection. Strip-mining is a highly effective means of spreading the infection. The organism invades the lung and, like TBC, is taken up by the macrophages causing a mild illness but resulting in a few granulomata which eventually will become calcified. Organisms are still present in the granulomata even when it becomes calcified and, if the patient becomes immunocompromised, are able to spread throughout the body. The diagnosis is made by finding antibodies to the organism in the blood or a positive skin test for the coccidiomycosis antigen.

Histoplasma capsulatum is also a fungus. It causes the disease "histoplasmosis." Like Valley Fever, the illness is usually a mild flu-like illness and like Valley Fever, the organism provokes the formation of granulomas in which it may survive awaiting to be reactivated and cause severe disease.

The organism is also found in the soil. Anyone who grew up in the Midwest will have a positive skin test for Histoplasmosis. It is also found in bird and bat droppings so that people who raise chickens, pigeons, and other birds as well as people who explore caves (spelunkers) will often contract the disease. Most people will not be aware that they had the disease, but the chest radiograph will show multiple small, calcified nodules as evidence of the prior infection.

Treatment for Histoplasmosis or Coccidiomycosis is rarely needed. In severe cases or cases in which the disease has become systemic or in patients who are immune incompetent because of medicines used to treat rheumatoid arthritis or systemic lupus erythematosus, potent therapy is available. The new agents are Itraconazole and Fluconazole. Itraconazole seems to perform better in skeletal lesions, whereas fluconazole performs better in pulmonary and soft tissue infection. Complications of both drugs include liver dysfunction.

Pneumocystis jiroveci (carinii) was a little-known organism that caused pneumonia in patients who had a renal transplant and were on immunosuppressant agents until the outbreak of AIDS in the 1970's. Suddenly with the advent of AIDS it became a quite common cause of an often-fatal pneumonia. It is a yeast-like fungus and not a bacteria or protozoan as was first suspected.

It invades the lungs of immune-compromised patients causing the Type 1 and Type 2 alveolar cells to "over replicate" filling the alveoli and damaging the alveolar lining. An intense and severe inflammatory reaction ensues, and the patient literally drowns in the fluid.

The organism usually causes an "atypical" pneumonia. The illness is characterized by a high fever, night sweats and progressively severe shortness of breath. The cough is usually mild and often non-productive. The chest x-ray shows an ARDS-like pattern although it can also show a lobar pneumonia or a patchy bronchial pneumonia. A pneumothorax is actually a common occurrence.

If the chest radiograph is normal, then a Gallium scan can be done. This test is positive 90% of the time. Arterial blood gases are often helpful. They will show that the hypoxia is far out of proportion to the findings on the chest x-ray. A sputum sample or a sample obtained on bronchoscopy will usually show the ring-like cystic organism which stains with a silver containing stain. Treatment is with Bactrim, a sulfa drug, or with Pentamidine. In both cases steroids are added to reduce the inflammation.

....

After the history and physical, the first step in **evaluating a patient with pneumonia** is to obtain a chest radiograph. This will tell the physician if there is an infiltrate consistent with pneumonia, whether it is focal like a lobar pneumonia, or diffuse like ARDS. If it is focal, its location will be helpful as well. Most typical pneumonias involve the lower lobes while some of the pneumonias we listed under the category "other" such as TBC or the fungal diseases involve the upper lobes or in the case of M. avium are associated with bronchiectasis. Some infections such as Pneumocystis can be associated with a pneumothorax or collapsed lung.

A simple blood count or CBC (complete blood count) must also be done. Most typical pneumonias are associated with a "leukocytosis" or elevated white cell count. The number of neutrophils are increased and often there are immature neutrophils called "bands" present. The atypical pneumonias or a very severe typical pneumonia may have a leukopenia or low WBC count.

Cultures of the blood should be done. A "sputum Gram stain, culture and sensitivity" are also done routinely. While these studies, unfortunately, are often not helpful, if by chance an organism is identified more specific treatment can be given. If an organism is found on the sputum culture it should be studied for its sensitivity to antibiotics.

The Gram stain dates back more than one hundred and forty years. The stain was developed by Hans Christian Gram, a Danish bacteriologist. It is based upon the fact that the cell walls of some bacteria contain much more of a chemical called peptidoglycan than others. Those bacteria with thick cell wall (especially the cocci) and lots of peptidoglycan take up a crystal violet dye avidly and hold onto it even when the slide is washed with alcohol. This gives them a deep blue color and they are called gram-positive. Those bacteria with a thin cell wall have only a small amount of peptidoglycan which is washed away with alcohol. Counterstaining these organisms with safranin gives them a pink color. These organisms are called gram-negative organisms.

Even in the outpatient setting, an oxygen saturation (using the co-oximeter) should be done. If the oxygen level is less than 92% hospitalization should be considered. Hospitalization should also be considered in patients with a rapid pulse or who have abnormal kidney function.

If the patient appears terribly ill, if hospitalization is being considered, or if the patient is already in the hospital, arterial blood gases should be done to determine the patient's oxygenation and acid-base status.

If one of the pneumonias listed under "other" is being considered, then sputum for acid fast bacilli and sputum for fungi should be done as well.

A urine sample should also be sent for the Legionella Antigen. This is the most effective means of diagnosing Legionnaires disease.

The **treatment** depends solely on whether a specific organism is identified or whether the pneumonia is a community acquired or hospital acquired pneumonia.

Vaccination plays a major role as well. All persons over the age of six months should have an influenza and RSV vaccination yearly. In addition, all persons over the age of 65 or who have underlying lung disease and are older than two should receive the pneumonia vaccine. The CDC recommends the pneumococcal polysaccharide vaccine (PPSV23 or Pneumovax which protects against 23 types of pneumococcal bacteria.

Seminars in Respiratory Disease

Suggestions for Minor Papers

1. Compare typical and atypical pneumonia
2. Compare the types of atypical pneumonias.
3. What kind of hospital equipment is contaminated by Pseudomonas and what can we do about it?
4. When is isolation important and what type of isolation is needed and why?
5. What is aspiration pneumonia and how is it treated?
6. When do we suspect a patient is immunocompetent and may have an unusual type of pneumonia?
7. What is a microbiome?
8. Discuss the different type of infectious disease precautions. Compare standard, contact, and aerosol precautions.
9. Compare covid, influenza, and RSV infection in the elderly

Peter A. Petroff, MD

Four

Pulmonary Artery Disease

Pulmonary Embolism and Pulmonary Hypertension

Pulmonary Arterial Disease is divided into two categories: acute pulmonary embolism and pulmonary artery hypertension. Acute pulmonary embolism (PE) is a most important killer. In the United States 100,000 people die each year from pulmonary embolism. Most of the deaths occur in hospitalized patients. Because of increasing awareness of the condition, the death rate appears to be decreasing. While patients in the hospital for both medical and surgical reasons have increased risk, patients with cancer, especially of the prostate, breast, and lung, as well as women who are pregnant or are on contraceptives, and patients who have inherited thrombotic disorders are at greatest peril. The mortality after a pulmonary embolism remains high, up to 30% in fact. Most patients die within the first week after an embolus due to a second pulmonary embolism or to shock. The death rate can be markedly reduced with effective anticoagulation. Clinical suspicion is the most effective means of lowering the death rate.

Over the last three decades Pulmonary Artery Hypertension (PH) has developed from a rare fatal disease affecting mainly young women into a large array of diseases, some common, some rare, which in total account for significant morbidity and pathology. There are now five classes of PH including primary disease of the pulmonary arteries, pulmonary hypertension due to left heart disease, pulmonary hypertension due to lung disease and hypoxemia, pulmonary hypertension due to chronic pulmonary emboli and a group of diseases in which the cause of the pulmonary hypertension remains elusive.

Treatment options have improved dramatically for each class of disease. But, like pulmonary embolism, clinical suspicion of the condition must be high in order to the make the diagnosis and begin the appropriate therapy.

Peter A. Petroff, MD

Case Presentations

1.

Max Z. is a 72-year-old Harley-Davidson biker. On the day of admission, he was riding his "hog" with his fellow bikers along a busy country highway. Somehow, he became separated from his friends. Out of the blue an SUV, travelling at extremely high speeds, sped passed him, forcing him off the road and into a ditch. The driver drove off without stopping. Max's friends saw the accident and called for help. An ambulance arrived within a few minutes and took him to the nearby community hospital.

Max was alert but had severe pain in his right leg, especially in the area around his hip. Otherwise, he felt, "as good as I should I guess."

The emergency physician saw Max immediately and did the initial history and physical. Max was a successful lawyer who founded a major law firm in the city. He was in his early 70's but remained active physically both biking and working out at the gym. He never smoked. He drank "moderately" which for Max meant three or four drinks a day. He had hypertension and took two medications to keep his blood pressure under control. He had no allergies. He had a cholecystectomy in the past. His mother died of a stroke when she was in her mid-fifties. His father is still alive. The family history was positive for hypertension and heart disease.

Max could not stand. He appeared to be about six feet tall and was moderately overweight. His temperature was 97 degrees F; his BP was 158/96; his pulse rate was 94.

His examination was unremarkable save for his right leg which showed a large amount of bruising about the right hip and upper femur. The right foot turned outwards, and any movement of the leg caused severe pain. Clearly, Max had a fracture of his femur. The doctor ordered x-rays of the right femur and hip as well as a CBC and chemistry profile.

The CBC showed a normal white cell count and platelet count, but the hemoglobin was decreased at 10.4 (normal is 14-18). The chemistry profile showed mildly abnormal liver enzymes, but the kidney function was normal. The x-rays showed a fracture at the neck of the femur.

The doctor advised Max that he needed to have surgery for the fracture, or he would never be able to walk. Max reluctantly agreed and was admitted to hospital. An orthopedic surgeon was called in for consultation. Surgery was planned for the next morning. In the meantime, Max was begun on IV fluids, and was fitted for intermittent pneumatic compression stockings on both his legs. The CBC would be repeated in four hours and again in the morning. An EKG was ordered as well as clotting studies including a protime and partial thromboplastin time.

The repeat CBC showed that the hemoglobin had decreased slightly to 9.7. The white count was stable, but the platelets had decreased from 300,000 to 170,000.

The surgery the next morning went well. Max was transferred to the ICU, more out of caution because of his age than any other reason. He was alert. His vital signs were normal. The doctor continued the intermittent compressive stockings and ordered incentive spirometry. He also began Max on low dose Lovenox, a blood thinner.

By the next morning Max felt "back to normal." After breakfast he was transferred to a private room on the orthopedic floor. The orthopedic surgeon told him that he had lost "a lot of blood." But he did not feel a transfusion was necessary at this point.

That evening, Max told the respiratory therapist that he was a little short of breath. He also had a pain in the right side of his chest. "It hurts to take even a little breath." The RT called the physician immediately who ordered a helical CAT scan of the chest. The CAT scan showed a clot in the artery to the right middle lobe as well as some mild generalized interstitial changes. The physician transferred Max back to the ICU and began therapeutic doses of Lovenox.

The following morning, Max was still more dyspneic. The doctor ordered blood gases, a CBC, and a chest radiograph.

The pO2 was 54 on room air, the pCO2 was 28, the pH was 7.56, and the HCO3 was 24. The WBC was 11.4, the hemoglobin was 9 gms, the platelet count was 75,000. The chest x-ray showed mild diffuse interstitial changes.

The doctor examined Max. He noticed a myriad of tiny red petechiae on his chest wall. His lungs showed a pleural friction rub and fine crackles over the right middle lobe. There was tenderness at the left calf with a positive Homan's sign. The doctor began Max on oxygen. He continued the Lovenox and the intermittent compression stockings.

That evening, Max became extremely short of breath. He was diaphoretic. His blood pressure was only 76/50 and his pulse was 126. The doctor ordered blood gases which showed the paO2 had fallen to 36. He intubated Max and placed him on a ventilator. The settings were an AC (assist control) of 12, TV of 540 cc (6 ccs/kg X 90 kg) and 100% oxygen. The paO2 rose to 125. The pCO2 was still in the low thirties. The Lovenox was continued. Sedation was needed to make Max comfortable with the low tidal volume setting.

Over the next forty-eight hours Max improved and was extubated on the third day. On a NC at 4 l/min his pO2 was now 86. The bedside chest radiograph was now clear. The petechiae had nearly completely resolved. A week later he was discharged on dabigatran or Pradaxa, a direct oral anticoagulant, and walked, with help, out of the hospital. His "hog" awaited him.

2.

Sandra K. came to the outpatient clinic at the University Health Center because she was short of breath. She had been to more than six physicians in the last two years. All of them told her, "It was all in my head."

She stated that she became aware of her symptoms two years before while she was going through a bitter divorce. She said she always ran two or three miles a day on the treadmill at the gym, but she had to stop because she "just couldn't do it anymore." She had no other symptoms. There was "no cough, no chest pain, no wheezing, nothing at all." The first doctor she saw examined her and took a chest radiograph. He told her everything was normal and gave her a prescription for an antidepressant. The other five doctors were no better. Now, she says, she has begun to lose weight and just walking a hundred feet is a chore. She is terribly afraid she will lose her job. "I'm a secretary so the work isn't physically hard, but I'm short of breath walking from the parking garage to the office."

She has never smoked; she does not drink. She doesn't take any medicines. "A few years ago, I took medicines to lose weight. I was nearly a hundred and fifty pounds, and I looked like a cow." The medicines didn't help her lose weight. They just made her jittery. She has no drug allergies, surgeries, or medical admissions. She is adopted.

She is 36 years of age. She is thin. Her height is 5'6" and her weight is 125 lbs. Her blood pressure and pulse are normal.

Examination of her head and neck is unremarkable but she is wearing a very bright red lipstick. The doctor asks her about her lipstick. "My lips are kind of bluish. If I don't wear lipstick I look like ghoulish." He smiled.

Her lungs were clear with good breath sounds. She lay down on the examination table with her head elevated at about 20 degrees. The doctor noted that her neck veins were distended. Examination of her heart showed a loud S2 (second heart sound) and a soft systolic ejection murmur just to the left of the sternum.

Her liver was enlarged to percussion, and she had slight pedal edema. The rest of the exam was normal.

The doctor ordered a chest radiograph, blood count, chemistry profile, ABGs and pulmonary function studies.

The Chest x-ray was normal. The blood count showed a hemoglobin of 18 grams. (Normal is 12-16). The chemistry profile was totally normal. The paO2 was 58, the pCO2 was 36, the pH was 7.48 and the HCO3 was 24. The pulmonary function studies are as follows:

Test	% of predicted
FVC	94%
FEV1	98%
TLC	94%
RV	96%
DCO	54%

The doctor reviewed the laboratory findings with Sandra. He said he wanted to do an echocardiogram and wanted her to see a cardiologist for a right heart catheterization. The echocardiogram showed that the right ventricle was enlarged and there was moderate tricuspid regurgitation. The estimated pulmonary artery pressure was 42 mm Hg at rest (the normal is less than 25 mm Hg). The heart catheterization confirmed these findings. When the cardiologist had Sandra inhale nitric oxide, the pressure in the pulmonary arteries dropped significantly.

The doctor diagnosed Sandra with type 1 pulmonary artery hypertension. She told the doctor she had indeed taken "fen-phen" for her weight. The doctor concluded this was the likely cause of her illness. He recommended she see the Pulmonary Hypertension Clinic.

The Clinic tested Sandra for several auto-immune diseases as well as for HIV infection. The tests were normal. Because she responded so well to nitric oxide, she was begun on diltiazem, a Calcium Channel Blocker. She returned in a month for follow-up. She reported that she was significantly better though she was still short of breath. She and the doctor discussed using several other medications including Viagra. However, Sandra wanted to wait a few months before deciding to take any additional medicines.

3.

Francesca C. is an extremely pleasant thirty-five-year-old woman who is getting more and more short of breath. She is consulting with the same pulmonologist she saw ten years ago. She relates her history as follows, "I don't know if you remember me. I saw you many years ago because I was short of breath. I was taking birth control pills and had a clot in my right leg that spread to my right lung. You found out that I was Factor V Leiden positive and began me on Coumadin. You may remember my mother died of a stroke when she was just 44 and my father died of a heart attack when he was sixty. My brother had a deep vein thrombosis in his leg when it was struck by a baseball. You said my history was quite convincing. The problem is that the shortness of breath never got better. In fact, it is getting much worse. I can't walk more than a hundred feet without stopping."

The doctor asked her if she was still taking her Coumadin. She said that she was, and her primary doctor checked her protime monthly and it was always in good range. She says she doesn't smoke or drink. She no longer takes the birth control pills. She is definitely not pregnant. "Can't happen," she says. She has no allergies. She has not had any surgery or medical admissions save for the admission with the pulmonary embolism. She works long hours as an illustrator, a job which she thoroughly enjoys.

She is five feet six inches and weighs one hundred and twenty pounds. Her blood pressure is 132/66 but her pulse is 102. Her oxygen saturation is 86%.

Her examination reveals her to be an alert, well-nourished woman in no acute distress while she is at rest. She is not cyanotic.

When she lies down with her head slightly elevated the doctor notices very prominent neck veins. Her lungs are clear with decreased breath sounds. Examination of her heart shows a grade 2/6 systolic ejection murmur best heard to the left of the sternum in the 2nd intercostal space.

Her liver is slightly enlarged but the spleen is not palpable. There is also trace pedal edema.

The doctor sends Francesca for laboratory studies, pulmonary function testing, and a chest radiograph.

The chest x-ray is normal. The CBC shows a hemoglobin of 16.7 (normal is 12-14). The white count and platelets are normal. The chemistry profile is normal. The protime shows an INR of 2.6 which is in therapeutic range. The pulmonary functions are as follows:

Vital Capacity	75% of normal
FEV1	75% of normal
FEV1/FVC	75%
MMF	75% of normal
TLC	75% of normal
RV	75% of normal
Diffusion Capacity	45% of normal

Francesca saw the doctor immediately after the pulmonary function testing. The doctor is concerned about pulmonary artery hypertension and orders an echocardiogram which confirms what he suspects. He tells her she needs to get additional studies. He discusses with her the two best options: a helical CAT scan of the lungs versus a ventilation-perfusion lung scan. After reviewing the pros and cons of both tests she agrees to get the ventilation-perfusion lung scan.

The V/Q lung scan shows matched and unmatched areas of ventilation and perfusion defects and is most consistent with chronic pulmonary emboli involving both lungs.

The doctor sends Francesca to a thoracic surgical center that specializes in the treating Type 4 Pulmonary Artery Hypertension. At the surgical center, a digital subtraction pulmonary angiogram is done which localizes the clots. Two weeks later she had surgery to remove the clots. The surgery takes more than six hours as clot after clot is removed from segmental arteries. She was on complete heart bypass for more than seven hours. She is sent to the ICU on a ventilator with partial arterial pressure support as well. Her hospital course is "stormy" but over the next two days she gradually improves. After nearly ten days in hospital, she is discharged to continue the blood thinner. She was changed from Coumadin to a direct thrombin inhibitor, Pradaxa.

Over the next two months her breathing improved.

Seminars in Respiratory Disease

Background for the presentations

These three cases represent a small part of the spectrum of pulmonary artery disease. The first case presents a patient with both a pulmonary embolism and fat embolism. The second case is a classic case of Type 1 chronic pulmonary artery hypertension, while the third case is a patient with chronic thromboembolic pulmonary hypertension or type 4 chronic pulmonary artery hypertension.

Important points

1. **Clinical suspicion** is the most important tool in order to make the diagnosis in all types of pulmonary vascular disease
2. **The primary symptom of a pulmonary embolism is shortness of breath.** Hemoptysis and chest pain occur in less than 30% of patients.
3. A pulmonary infarction occurs only when both the bronchial artery circulation and the pulmonary artery circulation are both impaired. In other words, the patient usually has a pulmonary embolism superimposed on congestive heart failure.
4. **Virchow's triad is hypercoagulability, endothelial injury, and immobilization.**
5. The most common cause of right heart failure is left heart failure.
6. The diffusing capacity is the most helpful pulmonary function in patients with pulmonary vascular disease. The diffusing capacity is reduced in most forms of pulmonary artery disease even if the rest of the PFTs are normal.
7. **Even one pulmonary embolism may result in Type 4 PAH**.
8. The treatment of Type 4 PAH is always surgical if the patient is able to tolerate the surgery. Otherwise the medicines used for treating Type 1 PAH can be tried.

Discussion

Pulmonary Embolism

Pulmonary vascular disease encompasses two large categories of disorders: pulmonary embolism (PE) and pulmonary artery hypertension (PAH). Pulmonary embolism tends to be an acute disease process whereas pulmonary artery hypertension tends to be a much more chronic disease, but there is definitely some overlap.

When we hear "pulmonary embolism" we think about grandma who died suddenly in her sleep two days after she had her gallbladder removed at St. Mary's in the Woods Hospital in Dayton, Ohio. But pulmonary embolism embraces a large number of pathologic processes.

What is an embolus? It is any tissue or substance that moves from one part of the body to another part of the body. We can say "Mom's breast cancer embolized to her brain" or "Dad's prostate cancer embolized to his spine." A pulmonary embolism is anything which moves to and blocks, completely or partially, a pulmonary artery, or any artery as a matter of fact. Certainly, the most common pulmonary embolism is a blood clot or thrombus. But fat can embolize. Fat is found in the bone marrow of the long bones. If the patient sustains a fractured hip, fat can be released form the bone marrow and travel to the lungs. If a patient has severe pancreatitis (inflammation of the pancreas) fat is released into the blood and can travel to the lungs. Another substance which can cause a pulmonary embolism is amniotic fluid which can be released from the uterus during the delivery of a baby.

We are all familiar with the murder mystery in which the nurse (never the doctor) injects air into a vein to kill someone. An air embolism is different from a pulmonary embolism, however, because the air ends up not in the lungs but instead fills the right ventricle. The right ventricle just can't pump air and the patient has a cardiac arrest.

When we think of a pulmonary embolism our first thought is most often a blood clot. Clotting is a normal part of the body's homeostasis. We do not want to die from a minor cut on our little finger of the left hand. On the other hand, clotting can also get out of control. We can have too much clotting, or we can have clots where there is no injury at all. Surgery activates the clotting pathway not just where the surgeon cut, but throughout the entire body! Deep vein thrombosis, a clot in a vein such as the femoral vein in the leg, occurs because of three factors: hypercoagulability, an endothelial injury (damaged blood vessel), and immobility. Together the three make up Virchow's Triad.

When there is an injury to the lining of a blood vessel (endothelium), two pathways are turned on immediately. The first is the formation of a platelet plug made up of activated platelets which first adhere to the damaged lining of the blood vessel, then change their shape producing long fingers or pseudopods. Then the platelets aggregate in bunches and secrete chemicals which in turn enhance the formation of thrombin. These chemicals include histamine, serotonin, fibrinogen, and several factors important in coagulation. Platelet clotting is impaired by aspirin and other nonsteroidal anti-inflammatory drugs.

The second pathway is found in the blood. It is the "clotting cascade" and it is also triggered by endothelial (the lining of the blood vessel) injury. The second pathway leads to the formation and propagation of a blood clot. The clotting cascade is made up of several proteins which when activated become enzymes which activate the next protein in the cascade. For example, when Factor XII becomes activated, it will become activated XII (or XIIa) which will catalyze the conversion of Factor XI into activated XI (or XIa). There are two separate pathways: the intrinsic and the extrinsic pathways. The intrinsic pathway is activated by exposure of the blood to a negatively charged surface. The extrinsic pathway, a more direct pathway, is activated by *tissue factor* (TF) or *tissue thromboplastin* released at the site of the injury by the damaged endothelial cells.

In the intrinsic pathway, contact with the negatively charged molecule results in the activation of Factor XII, which then activates Factor XI, which then activates Factor IX, and which finally activates both Factor VIII and X. In the extrinsic pathway, TF directly activates Factor VII which then activates Factor X. It is the activated Factor X which then activates *prothrombinase* which converts prothrombin to thrombin which, at last, converts fibrinogen to fibrin forming the clot. Studies on rabbits show the clot begins forming within minutes and the thrombus is fully formed by the third day after an injury.

Balancing the clot formation process is the clot dissolution process. After the clot has formed and the bleeding has stopped, the clot must be reabsorbed. If not, the thrombus can propagate and damage uninjured tissue. Protein C, Protein S and Factor V are all necessary to terminate clot formation. Together they inactivate the activated Factor V and VIII, turning off the coagulation cascade. If they are deficient, clotting will occur with minimal trauma. Factor V Leiden is an abnormal Factor V which cannot be inactivated by Protein C. Thus, it will cause a hypercoagulable state as shown in our second patient. In addition, if Protein C or Protein S is absent the patient will be hypercoagulable as well. The last step in dissolving a clot occurs when plasminogen is converted to plasmin by the endothelial cells, which cleaves the fibrin and fibrinogen leading to dissolution of the clot.

Pulmonary embolism accounts for about 24% of deaths at community hospitals. It is the third most common cardiovascular cause of death after acute myocardial infarction and stroke. About 100,000 Americans die of a pulmonary embolism yearly. Those numbers have been nearly constant for the last sixty years. In 2006, 247,000 patients were discharged from nonfederal, short-stay hospitals in the United States with a diagnosis of a pulmonary embolism. Large or fatal pulmonary embolisms are found at autopsy in 5-10% of hospitalized patients and small pulmonary embolisms in about 40-50%. Most (80%) of the pulmonary emboli found at autopsy were unsuspected when the patient was alive.

Deep vein thromboses are clots that form in the large veins. More than half form in the calf and about a third form in the thigh. Clots in the veins of the upper extremity are much less common. In 2012, more than a half-million adults were hospitalized with deep vein thrombosis.

Typically, a patient is admitted to hospital with trauma, a medical condition such as congestive heart failure, or for a scheduled surgery. Then two or three days after admission, he or she has a pulmonary embolism. Almost all pulmonary emboli originate in the legs as deep vein thrombosis (DVT). The symptoms of a DVT include painful swelling in the calf or thigh. Sometimes the skin over the clot will be inflamed. Most of the time there are no symptoms or signs. The patient just presents with a pulmonary embolism.

An acute pulmonary embolism can be categorized as massive, sub-massive, and low risk. Massive pulmonary embolism is associated with **hypotension and even shock** and carries a 25-50% mortality rate. The treatment is to immediately start intravenous heparin as well as considering interventional therapy including thrombolytics, embolectomy, and VA ECMO. Most physicians now favor immediate thrombectomy via a right heart catheterization.

The pulmonary embolism can be described as "submassive" when the patient is stable clinically but has right ventricular heart failure (cor pulmonale). These patients have a 3-8% mortality rate. The right ventricular failure is diagnosed either by a CAT scan or by Echocardiogram and the treatment is similar to patients with a massive pulmonary embolism. The low-risk patients respond well to anticoagulation alone.

A pulmonary embolism can also be classified by its location. If it is located in the main pulmonary artery with branches into both the left and right main stem arteries, it is a *Saddle Embolism*. If the PE blocks a lobar artery, it is a *lobar embolism*. If it blocks a segment of the lung, it is a *segmental embolism*. A saddle embolism is found in about 5% of patients with a PE.

Who is likely to get a PE? Any patient who is hospitalized and is immobilized is a candidate for a pulmonary embolism. But there are factors which increase the risk substantially: patients with cancer especially prostate, lung and breast cancer, patients who are pregnant or who are on contraceptives, patients who have had trauma or who are undergoing surgical procedures, patients with strokes, patients with congestive heart failure and finally patients who have deficiency of Protein C or S or who have Factor V Leiden.

What is the pathophysiology of a pulmonary embolism? The clot blocks an artery cutting off perfusion to the distal alveoli. This results in an increase in dead space ventilation. In addition, the clot activates the inflammatory pathways resulting in the release of chemicals such as serotonin that cause bronchoconstriction resulting in areas of relative shunting. Thus ventilation/perfusion inequality is profoundly worsened resulting in hypoxemia. The blocked arteries raise the pressure in the pulmonary artery and can, if the blockage is severe enough, cause acute right heart failure or cor pulmonale. Finally, in some patients, especially those with congestive heart failure, the lung tissue distal to the obstruction will die. This is called a **pulmonary infarction**. The patient with a pulmonary infarction is the patient who develops chest wall pain or pleurisy and is found on physical examination to have a pleural friction rub.

The most common symptom of a pulmonary embolism is shortness of breath. It is found in up to 97% of patients. An inpatient who suddenly develops shortness of breath must always be suspected of having a pulmonary embolism. Less common symptoms include cough, chest wall pain like pleurisy, and hemoptysis. These are found in only about a third of patients. Finally, some patients will present with syncope or even a sudden cardiac arrest.

Physical signs are just as allusive. Most patients have only dyspnea and tachycardia. A few, with moderate size pulmonary emboli will have a loud second heart sound, best heard in the 2nd left intercostal space adjacent to the sternum. They may also have an exceptionally soft S3 heard to the right of the sternum due to right ventricular failure and tricuspid insufficiency. Still fewer patients have massive pulmonary emboli. They may show frank signs of cor pulmonale with neck vein distention, a large liver, and slight pedal edema.

Signs of a DVT such as redness, tenderness or swelling in a calf, occur in one in ten patients with a pulmonary edema. If the patient has had a pulmonary infarction, then crackles may be heard over the infarct and sometimes a pleural rub as well. A pleural rub sounds like two pieces of leather being rubbed together.

What was true when I was in medical school is still true today. The patient usually doesn't die from the first clot to his or her lungs; it is the second one that gets them. Thus, if the diagnosis can be made early on, the patient will walk out of the hospital; if not, he will be carried out on a gurney. What this means is that if you suspect a pulmonary embolism, you must treat the patient while you set about doing diagnostic testing.

One of the simplest tests to apply to a hospitalized patient with shortness of breath is the Well's criteria: If there are clinical signs and symptoms of a DVT the patient gets 3 points. If there are no other disorders that could be the cause of the symptoms the patient gets 3 points. If the heart rate is greater than 100, the patient gets 1.5 points. If the patient has been immobilized for 3 days or more or has had surgery in the past 4 weeks, the patient gets 1.5 points. If the patient has a prior history of a proven pulmonary embolism, the patient gets 1.5 points. If the patient coughs up blood, he gets 1 point and lastly if the patient has been treated for cancer in the last six months, he gets a point. All the points are added together. If the score is less than 4, a pulmonary embolism is unlikely and there is only a 3% risk of a pulmonary embolism.

If a pulmonary embolism is considered unlikely, then a D-dimer can be helpful. The D-dimer test measures the breakdown products of fibrin, the protein that makes up the clot. If the sensitive D-dimer is within normal range for your hospital, then a PE is very unlikely. If it is positive, the patient may have a PE, but false positives occur in anyone who has had trauma, surgery, is pregnant, has an inflammatory disease such as Rheumatoid Arthritis or has cancer. **Thus, the test is only helpful if it is negative.**

A chest x-ray is almost always done. It is generally normal. Occasionally, if the patient has had a pulmonary infarct, there may be focal atelectasis or infiltrate, or a pleural based cone-shaped lesion referred to as a Hampton Hump. The diaphragm may be elevated on the affected side.

An electrocardiogram should be done as well. This may show signs of right heart strain or a new arrhythmia such as atrial fibrillation or atrial flutter, all of which makes a PE more likely. Most often, the EKG shows only tachycardia. Certainly, ABGs should be done. They may show hypoxemia with a mild respiratory alkalosis, but hypoxemia does not need to be present. However, a patient can have an O2 saturation greater than 90% and still have a PE.

Rather than getting a chest x-ray, the first step could be a Helical CAT scan (Computed Tomographic Angiography (CTA)) of the chest. A high-speed CAT scan is done while the patient is given a bolus of iodine containing contrast material which will light up all the blood vessels of the lungs. A pulmonary artery that is "cut off" is diagnostic. Sometimes the clot can actually be visualized. The Helical CAT scan is now the gold standard for making the diagnosis.

If the patient is allergic to iodine, is pregnant, or is unwilling to take a CAT scan of the chest then a ventilation/perfusion lung scan can be done. In this test, the patient is given a dose of radioactive albumin intravenously. The albumin is a protein of sufficient size to become lodged in the small capillaries of the lung. A Geiger counter device then scans the chest. If the patient is normal, there will be a homogeneous uptake of the albumin. If the patient has a blood clot or pneumonia, there will be an area that does not take up the albumin. In that case the patient inhales radioactive Xenon and the study is repeated. A patient with a pulmonary embolism will have relatively normal airways so the uptake will be homogeneous. If the patient has pneumonia there will be a matched defect, meaning both perfusion and ventilation are absent in the suspicious area. The ventilation/perfusion lung scan can be negative (normal perfusion), positive (abnormal perfusion with normal ventilation) or indeterminate (a matching defect). Most tests end up being indeterminate unfortunately, but two or more indeterminate areas make a pulmonary embolism more likely.

If the CTA cannot be done and the ventilation/perfusion lung scan is indeterminate, then an ultrasound of the legs should be done looking for DVT's. This is sometimes helpful. The other alternative is to do a localized pulmonary angiogram. The patient essentially has a catheter placed in the area of the lung that was abnormal on the ventilation/perfusion lung scan. Iodine is injected just to the area in question. This test is often diagnostic.

Most patients with a pulmonary embolism can be diagnosed with appropriate testing. Some cannot and in those circumstances, the clinician needs to make a decide based solely on his suspicions whether the patient should be treated.

If the patient is acutely short of breath or is hypotensive, an echocardiogram must be done to determine if there is right heart strain or findings consistent with pulmonary artery hypertension. This study needs to be done as soon as possible. If the patient has signs of right heart failure, more aggressive therapy including the use of V-A ECMO perfusion, or immediate use of thrombolytic agents to dissolve the clot will be called for.

Treatment involves either removing the clot directly or "thinning the blood." The most important first step is always heparin, either unfractionated given IV or fractionated (low molecular weight) given subcutaneously. Heparin inactivates thrombin stopping thrombin from converting fibrinogen into fibrin. It is a large polysaccharide that binds to antithrombin III (AT) which changes the shape of the AT molecule so that it inactivates thrombin much more quickly than normal.

An oral blood thinner is started at the same time as the heparin. Coumadin works by stopping the vitamin K dependent synthesis of Factors II, VII, IX, and X in the liver. The direct anticoagulants (DAOC) are the newest class of medications, but they have already become the standard of care. Dabigatran works by inhibiting Thrombin while Apixaban and Rivaroxaban work by inhibiting activated Factor X, which is the Factor that activates Thrombin. The main problem with the DAOC's is their much higher cost compared to Coumadin.

If the patient has a massive pulmonary embolism with shock, then the patient should be placed on an ECMO (extracorporeal membrane oxygenation) machine with the venous line placed in the right atrium and the blood returned to the arterial side. It turns out that massive pulmonary embolism causes acute right heart failure. The abrupt rise in pulmonary artery pressure "stuns" the heart. The heart can take days to weeks to recover. ECMO bypasses the heart completely allowing time for the heart to heal while maintaining the patient's oxygenation.

Lastly, if the patient has a pulmonary embolism while he is on a blood thinner, then a Greenfield filter can be placed in the inferior vena cava to prevent further clots from reaching the lungs.

How long does a patient need to remain on anticoagulants? If the patient has a reason for the clot and has no family history of a clotting disorder, then the patient should be treated for three months. If, on the other, the clot occurred for little or no reason, or the patient has a family history of clotting, or if he or she is deficient in Protein C or S or has Factor V Leiden, then he or she will need to be on anticoagulants forever.

Can we prevent clotting in the hospital? We can certainly try. We can give low dose fractionated heparin (Lovenox) subcutaneously. Coumadin can also be used. Finally, intermittent compressive stockings or leggings are used, but they are not as effective as low molecular weight heparin.

There is one syndrome that bridges acute pulmonary embolism and chronic pulmonary artery hypertension. This is the patient with multiple recurrent pulmonary emboli occurring over months or years. The patient presents with shortness of breath and signs of cor pulmonale. The chest x-ray will show large pulmonary arteries and mild interstitial changes, patchy atelectasis, or areas of pneumonia. The EKG will show right heart strain. The diagnosis is made by the helical CAT scan of the chest (CTA) and the treatment is life-time anticoagulation.

The symptoms and signs of a **fat embolism** are a far cry from those of blood clots. Fat embolism behaves more like the acute respiratory distress syndrome than a typical blood clot. Fat globules are found throughout the pulmonary circulation and enter the systemic system as well causing the fat embolism syndrome (FES) which consists of hypoxemia, neurologic abnormalities and a petechial rash often involving the conjunctiva and the anterior chest wall. The hypoxemia can be quite severe. One half of patients with a long bone fracture who develop fat emboli will require ventilator support. The neurologic symptoms include confusion, seizures, and even focal neurological defects.

Supporting laboratory findings include thrombocytopenia, anemia, and hypocalcemia. Coagulation abnormalities may be present as well. The chest radiograph is usually normal though a pattern consistent with ARDS may be seen. The diagnosis is made on clinical findings only. Invasive studies need not be done as there is no specific therapy. Supportive therapy is the key. Steroids and heparin have been tried in the past, but they have not been proven to be helpful.

Chronic Pulmonary Hypertension

Chronic Pulmonary Hypertension (PH) is far less common than pulmonary emboli but like pulmonary embolism the disease is fatal if not treated. While the incidence of PH is low compared to the incidence of PE, more than 70 million people in America are "at risk" for developing the disorder because they have heart disease or lung disease or one of the other known causes of PH. Pulmonary hypertension is a chronic, progressive, and incurable disease involving the pulmonary arteries and right heart. It is defined as a resting pulmonary artery pressure greater than 25 mm Hg. The normal resting pulmonary artery pressure is less than 15 mm Hg. Several different classes of diseases can result in PH. What they have in common is that each type of disease causes pulmonary hypertension, and each class of disease causes right heart failure. But each of them has its own pathophysiology and each class includes a myriad of disorders. A simple summary is a good place to start:

1. Class 1   PAH or primary pulmonary artery hypertension
2. Class 2   PH due to left ventricular heart disease
3. Class 3   PH due to lung disease with hypoxia
4. Class 4   chronic thromboembolic pulmonary hypertension
5. Class 5   conditions causing PH that have unknown pathogenesis

Although each class of disease has its own features, certain characteristics are seen throughout all the groups. Patients with PH almost always complain of shortness of breath and fatigue even before they have problems with gas exchange. In addition, the patient may have chest pain similar in quality to patients with angina. The pain is usually a crushing substernal pain elicited by exercise and relieved by rest. The pain is believed to be due to right ventricular ischemia. The second heart sound in the pulmonic area (2nd left parasternal interspace) is often quite loud and there may be murmurs of tricuspid regurgitation and pulmonic regurgitation though these murmurs are exceedingly difficult to hear. Lastly there may be a right ventricular S3 or an S4 similar to the "gallops" heard from the left ventricle during left ventricular failure.

The diagnostic workup begins with the chest radiograph which may show large pulmonary arteries and right ventricular hypertrophy. In the case of Class 1 PAH, there may be large pulmonary arteries with pruning of the smaller arterial branches. The second step is always an echocardiogram which will confirm the presence of a thickened right ventricular wall with right ventricular failure as well as show signs of pulmonary hypertension. A right heart catheterization must then be done to measure the pressure in the pulmonary artery, measure the left atrial pressure or wedge pressure, and lastly determine if the patient has significant improvement after being given nitric oxide.

Class 1 PH is due to disease of the arteries and arterioles of the lung itself. In this disease, the pulmonary artery pressure is high while the wedge pressure or left ventricular end diastolic pressure (LVEDP) is normal. The resistance of the pulmonary artery is equal to the difference between pulmonary artery pressure and the wedge pressure which is then divided by the cardiac output.

pulmonary artery resistance = (Pulmonary artery pressure – wedge pressure)/cardiac output

The pulmonary artery resistance must be increased in patients with Class 1 PH.

In patients with type 1 PH, the lining of the blood vessels become thickened and the smooth muscle in the wall of even the smallest arteriole becomes hypertrophied. The microscopic pathognomonic finding is the presence of a "web-like" structure in the small muscular arteries. These are tiny vascular channels within the lumen of arteries in which in situ thrombosis has occurred. Thrombosis and inflammation are always present. The endothelial lining of the tiny pulmonary arterioles produces **increased** amounts of both serotonin and endothelin, which are vasoconstrictors and cause inflammation, and **decreased** amounts of nitric oxide which is a vasodilator. The underlying mechanism appears to have to do with **mitochondrial failure**. Normally, glucose is broken down to two molecules of pyruvate with the release of two ATPs per molecule of sugar. The pyruvate then enters the mitochondria to be metabolized into CO_2 and H_2O and 36 molecules of ATP (the aerobic pathway). Oxygen is needed for the latter reaction to occur. If there is hypoxia, the pyruvate is converted to lactic acid and excreted. Patients who have cancer and patients who have type 1 PH behave as if they are hypoxic. The mitochondria do not metabolize the pyruvate. Little ATP is produced, and the tissues become energy starved. This likely triggers the inflammatory pathway in the endothelial cells.

The disease can be idiopathic (IPAH) or it can occur as part of another disease process. Idiopathic pulmonary arterial hypertension is inherited in 10% of patients in which case it is called heritable pulmonary arterial hypertension (HPAH). The disorders that can cause Class 1 PH include the autoimmune or connective tissue diseases such as scleroderma and rheumatoid arthritis, cirrhosis of the liver, HIV infection, and exposure to certain chemicals, especially the weight loss chemicals aminorex and fenfluramine (phen-fen).

About eighty percent of the patients with IPAH are women in their thirties and forties. They present with unexplained dyspnea, fatigue and even syncope. On average it takes two years before a doctor makes the correct diagnosis. Untreated IPAH is always fatal with a life expectancy of just two or three years after diagnosis. However, recently, several new therapies have become available. The oldest of these are the calcium channel antagonists, especially Nifedipine and Diltiazem. These drugs are only indicated in patients whose pulmonary artery pressures become normal after nitric oxide inhalation, so their use is quite limited. In those patients who have at least a partial response to nitric acid four classes of vasodilators are now used:

1. Prostacyclin derivatives: epoprostenol is given by continuous intravenous injection through a permanently implanted central venous catheter using a portable infusion pump. It is considered the first line therapy in patients with severe disease because of its efficacy. The drug has been shown to improve functional capacity and survival. Ilolprost, another prostacyclin, is given by inhalation using a special nebulizer. Its disadvantage is that it must be given at least six times a day.
2. Endothelin-1 receptor blockers: Endothelin is a potent vasoconstrictor responsible in part for the inflammation seen in PAH and scleroderma. Bosentan is a non-selective endothelin receptor blocker which has been shown to improve exercise capacity. It is given orally.
3. Phosphodiesterase inhibitors (PDE5 Inhibitors) prolong the vasodilatory effect of nitric oxide. Sildenafil (Viagra) has been shown to improve exercise capacity in patients with group 1 PAH.
4. Guanylate cyclase stimulators increase the sensitivity of the nitric oxide receptor to nitric oxide and also stimulate the receptor causing vasodilation directly. They

are used in both Class 1 PH as well as in Class 4 PH (Chronic thromboembolic pulmonary hypertension).

Patients with IPAH are also treated with blood thinners to decrease the risk of thrombosis occurring in a pulmonary artery or arteriole, although this practice is still considered controversial.

Class 2 PH is due to left heart failure. **Left sided heart failure is the most common cause of pulmonary hypertension and right heart failure.** The chest radiograph is often helpful to identify patients with Class 2 PH. The heart is enlarged with systolic heart failure (though it may be normal in size with diastolic heart failure), there is cephalization of blood flow (redistribution of blood flow to the upper zones of the lung), there is often interstitial and alveolar edema and, much less commonly, Kerley B lines. The echocardiogram will usually establish the diagnosis showing signs of left ventricular disease, either an elevated LVEDV or a markedly thickened left ventricular wall. The treatment is directed at the underlying heart disease, although in some cases, vasodilators may be tried.

Class 3 PH is due to lung disease and hypoxia. This is the second most common cause of pulmonary hypertension. Chronic bronchitis, asthma, sleep apnea and neurologic diseases which affect respiration will cause hypoxia and hypoxemia. Hypoxia is the main culprit causing the pulmonary hypertension though respiratory acidosis and secondary polycythemia may also play a minor role. Hypoxia and a low pH both cause vasoconstriction resulting in elevated pulmonary artery pressures. In addition, emphysema and pulmonary interstitial lung disease destroy not only the alveoli but also the surrounding capillary blood vessels. The treatment of this type of PH is to treat the underlying lung disease and to correct the hypoxia and hypoxemia.

Class 4 PH is chronic thromboembolic pulmonary hypertension (CTEPH). Patients with this disorder present with dyspnea and fatigue often without a history of ever having a pulmonary embolism or DVT. Usually, the patient has had several pulmonary embolisms occurring over the years but even one pulmonary embolism can result in the disease. Because there is extensive scarring of the lung due to the organized intra-arterial clots, anticoagulants are generally not very helpful. The treatment is the surgical removal of the clots. Unlike a pulmonary embolus where the diagnosis is best made with CTA (computer tomographic angiography), a lung scan is the diagnostic tool of choice. Recently, a new medication, Adempas or Rociguat, was introduced to treat both Class 4 PAH and some cases of class 1 PAH. The drug is a soluble guanylate cyclase stimulant which increases the production of cyclic guanyl monophosphate (cyclic GMP). As you recall from the lecture on asthma cyclic GMP is a bronchoconstrictor, but it *also dilates the pulmonary arteries*. It does this by both a direct action on the arteries as well as making the arteries more sensitive to nitric oxide. It is nitric oxide which normally stimulates the endogenous production of cyclic GMP. In some patients with PAH nitric oxide is reduced. In clinical studies, Adempas lowered the pulmonary artery resistance and increased the exercise capacity of patients with PAH. Side effects include gastrointestinal upset and headache but serious side effects such as hemoptysis have occurred as well. The drug can't be taken with medications including sildenafil and sildenafil-like agents, nitrates, and theophyllines.

Class 5 PH are those conditions associated with pulmonary artery hypertension which have an unknown pathophysiology. Several hematologic diseases are in this group, as is Sarcoidosis. In all cases, the therapy is directed at the underlying cause.

Suggestions for minor papers

1. Compare the classic pulmonary function of patients with chronic bronchitis, interstitial fibrosis, and pulmonary embolism.
2. Discuss the importance of the six-minute walk in following patients with PH.
3. What is the relationship between pulmonary emboli and chronic thromboembolic pulmonary artery hypertension?
4. How does hypoxia cause pulmonary artery hypertension?
5. What is the role of the respiratory therapist in the diagnosis and treatment of a pulmonary embolism?
6. What is the WHO functional class?
7. What is the fat embolism syndrome?

Peter A. Petroff, MD

Five

Acute Respiratory Distress Syndrome

The acute respiratory distress syndrome (ARDS) is a pulmonary disease defined by the presence of hypoxemia and diffuse but patchy pulmonary interstitial changes on the chest radiographs or CAT scans of the lung in the presence of a trauma or any illness capable of causing the disorder.

The disease is a very old disease. During the World Wars it was called "shock lung." During the Viet Nam War it was called "Da Nang Lung." When I worked at the Burn Unit at Fort Sam Houston during the Viet Nam era, we called it "Burn Lung Syndrome." The syndrome, first described in the late-1960's, was initially called the "Adult Respiratory Distress Syndrome" to distinguish it from "Hyaline Membrane Disease" of the newborn because pathologically the two conditions are quite similar in appearance and even clinical presentation. In both conditions the alveoli are filled with a blue staining, proteinaceous "hyaline membrane."

ARDS is a syndrome encompassing conditions as diffuse as "fat embolism syndrome," septic shock, and influenza. They are all bound together by the common pathophysiology of increased permeability of the pulmonary capillary and alveolar endothelium so that proteins and even red blood cells can leak from the capillary to the interstitial tissues and then into the alveoli. In congestive heart failure the pulmonary edema fluid is low in protein. In ARDS the fluid that fills the alveoli is high in protein and fibrin and stains blue with a common dye, hence the name "hyaline membrane disease." The Alveolar Type One cells are damaged and the Alveolar Type Two cells hypertrophy replacing the damaged alveolar lining cells.

The overall survival rate for ARDS is about 40%, but with the advent of advanced respiratory care, it is generally not the lung disease that kills the patient. Rather it is either the underlying condition or the development of secondary organ failure, especially sepsis, as well as liver and renal failure.

Peter A. Petroff, MD

Case Presentations

1.

Ann C. is a 38-year-old woman, mother of three, who was found by her husband the morning of admission lying in a pool of blood and barely responsive. He called 911 immediately. When they arrived, she was diaphoretic and unresponsive. Her blood pressure was 76 systolic. Her pulse was 126. The EMS technicians placed an oral pharyngeal tube and began her on 100% oxygen. They also started IV fluids (5% D/NS) at 250 cc an hour. The patient was transferred to the hospital ER within just a few minutes.

In the ER, the physician intubated the patient, placed her on a ventilator with 100% O2 and AC of 12 with a TV of 600 cc. He did not add any PEEP because of her extremely low blood pressure. He then obtained a "stat" chest radiograph, ABGs. CBC, and chemistry profile.

The chest x-ray showed the endotracheal tube was in good position and the patient's lungs were "clear." The CBC showed a hemoglobin of 7 gm/100cc. (Normal is 12-16 gm/100cc). The WBC was 2,000 with more than 25% bands (premature neutrophils). ABGs on 100% oxygen showed a paO2 of 140, a pCO2 of 32 a pH of 7.24 and a HCO3 of 16. The PaO2/fiO2 ratio was 140/1.00 or 140 indicating severe hypoxemia.

The blood pressure remained in the 70's and the doctor ordered a dopamine drip as well as a "type and cross" for four units of blood.

The doctor then got some history from the husband. Ann had found out she was 3 months pregnant. She went to family planning but was told that it was against the law for them to recommend someone who do an abortion. They lived in a rural area not far from the border and one of her neighbors knew someone who knew someone who could help. She crossed the border and had an abortion. At first the doctor tried oral medicine. When that did not work, the "doctor" removed the fetus as well as he could. On her way back across the border she began bleeding. She also vomited the night before admission and became so weak she could barely stand but she refused to go to the hospital. The husband thought it was mostly out of shame and the fear of prosecution.

Ann did not smoke or drink. She did not take any medicines and had no drug allergies. She had no other surgery or medical admissions. All three of her prior deliveries were vaginal. Her examination was largely unremarkable save for her pallor and mottling of her skin. Her abdomen was distended and when the doctor touched it gently the patient winced.

A stat CAT scan was done which showed the uterine wall was perforated. There was free air throughout the abdomen. The doctor called a gynecologist to see her. The gynecologist said he would see her in the surgical suite and the patient was transferred upstairs for immediate surgery. Additional laboratory studies were done looking for a bleeding disorder.

The gynecologist did a complete hysterectomy under light anesthesia. The blood arrived as the case was finishing. The anesthesiologist placed a large bore intravenous catheter and a central line. He infused blood through both lines. By the time she was in recovery her blood pressure had increased to 90 systolic. The dopamine, blood and IV fluids were continued. Blood cultures were done. The patient was begun on Fortaz and Cipro and she was transferred to the surgical intensive care unit (SICU).

Her blood pressure slowly improved over the next two hours. The dopamine was weaned. The doctor added 5 cm. of PEEP and repeated the ABGs on admittance to the SICU. The PaO2 was 85, the pCO2 was 36, the pH was 7.45 and the HCO3 was up to 22. The patient was still unresponsive.

The following morning, the PaO2 was 64, the pCO2 was 32, the pH was 7.52 and the HCO3 was 24. The Chest x-ray now showed diffuse interstitial infiltrates in both lung fields. The renal function had deteriorated. The creatinine went from a normal 0.76 to 1.6 indicating the kidneys had completely stopped working. The hemoglobin was now up to 12 mg/100cc. The blood pressure was 124/82 and the pulse rate 92. The PEEP was increased to 10 and a nephrologist (renal specialist) was called to see the patient.

The IV fluids were tapered to prevent fluid overload. The anesthesiologist inserted a Swan-Ganz catheter through the central line. The wedge pressure was 22 indicating the patient was likely already fluid overloaded. Lasix was given, strict intake and output monitoring was continued.

The following morning, the chest x-ray was worse. There were still more infiltrates. The creatinine had climbed to 2.5 again indicating the kidneys were still shut down. The wedge pressure was still 20. The blood gases were stable. At 3 in the afternoon the patient had a cardiac arrest and died. The husband refused to allow an autopsy to be done.

2.

Roger Z, a 40-year-old-male, was admitted to the emergency room with fever, chills, night sweats, generalized weakness, and a severe cough productive of scanty phlegm. He had been ill for 5 days. The illness began with generalized aches and pains and a low-grade fever. He thought it was the flu. He never got a "flu shot." He did not believe in them. In the last 24 hours, however, he became much more toxic. His temperature spiked; he began having shaking chills; the cough kept him awake all night.

He was a non-smoker. He drank one or two beers a week. He took Vasotec for his blood pressure. He was allergic to sulfa medicines. He has never had surgery nor been admitted to hospital before. His family history was non-contributory.

His physical exam revealed bluish lips and fingertips. He was short of breath just transferring from cart to cart. His temperature was 102 degrees F. His BP was 148/92. His weight was 150 lbs. His pulse was 124. Examination of his head and neck showed mild pharyngitis. His lungs showed diffuse inspiratory crackles. The examination of his heart, abdomen and extremities was normal.

The chest x-ray showed mild diffuse interstitial changes. The radiologist said, "Nothing to write home about." The blood count was normal as were the liver and kidney tests. Serology for influenza was positive. The doctor ordered blood gases. The paO2 was 76, the pCO2 was 28, the HCO3 was 24 and the pH was 7.5. The A-a O2 gradient was {150 – (1.25 X 28)} – 76 or 39 which is quite high. Normal is about 5-10 mm Hg. Even though the patient's pO2 was 76 he had a markedly abnormal A-a O2 gradient.

The doctor admitted Roger to the medical intensive care unit. He began him on oxygen at 2 liters/min per nasal cannula. He also began Tamiflu and Relenza to treat the influenza. The patient was begun on IV fluids as well. Over the next 12 hours, Roger's O2 saturation dropped to 88%. The doctor intubated Roger and placed him on a ventilator set at Assist Control of 12, TV of 500, 60% O2 and PEEP of 5. The ABGs were repeated in one hour. The pO2 was 104, the pCO2 was 36, the HCO3 was 24, and the pH was 7.42. The settings were continued. Roger's vital signs remained normal. His temperature returned to normal by the next morning. The morning blood gases were markedly improved. The patient was extubated that afternoon. He went home two days later.

3.

Jun B. was a 78-year-old male who was brought to the emergency room by his wife Linda, a physician, because of cough and fever. She had been exposed to the Coronavirus two weeks earlier on hospital rounds. Though she felt completely well, she was tested for the virus four days after her exposure and tested positive. She tried to isolate herself from her husband as much as possible when she got the news. She was fearful for him because he had had heart surgery several years before. Two days before admission, Jun told his wife that he lost his sense of smell and taste. She took him to his doctor the same day. Everyone in the office, including doctors, staff, and patients were wearing masks. The doctor sent him for a screening test for the Coronavirus and advised the Jun and Linda that he should remain at home unless he developed a fever or cough. If he developed either symptom he should go at once to the emergency room.

The next day, Jun had a mild irritating dry cough. The cough was mild but incessant. He also felt tired and had diffuse muscle aches. He took an over-the-counter cough medicine but was not able to sleep that night. The doctor called Jun to let him know that he had the virus. The following day, the morning of admission, Jun developed a fever to 101 degrees. Linda called an ambulance and Jun was taken to the emergency room at the University Hospital, which still had a few beds in the ICU.

Precautions to prevent the spread of the virus were widespread. All the nurses, doctors and respiratory therapists wore gowns, N-95 masks with eye shields and gloves. All the equipment was frequently disinfected. Standard, contact, and airborne precautions were strictly enforced.

In the emergency room, Jun had a temperature of 101. He was alert, diaphoretic, and dyspneic. His vital signs showed a blood pressure of 146/94 and a pulse rate of 124. The EKG monitor showed that he was in sinus rhythm.

Jun gave his history to the doctor including the results of the screening for the Coronavirus. His main symptom still was his cough and loss of his sense of smell. He did not have nausea or diarrhea. He worked with his wife in her office and sometimes made rounds with her in the hospital. He was her accountant and office manager. He smoked in the past, having quit when he had his heart attack ten years before. He did not drink. He took Toprol, a Beta blocker for his heart, Lipitor for his cholesterol, a baby aspirin, as well as a multivitamin. He had no drug allergies. He was active, walking two miles a day. His family history was positive for heart disease and diabetes. The doctor ordered a chest radiograph, CBC, chemistry profile, ABGs, urinalysis, EKG, BNP, C-reactive protein, d-dimer. and troponin levels. He began Jun on oxygen at 2l/min.

The CXR showed fluffy infiltrates in both lower lobes. The ABGs showed a pO2 of 58, a pCO2 of 28, a pH of 7.48 and a HCO3 of 24. The CBC showed that the neutrophils were increased while the lymphocytes were decreased. The chemistry profile showed a mild increase in the liver enzymes, but the kidney tests were normal. The urinalysis was normal while the EKG showed only signs of the old myocardial infarction. There were no acute changes. The troponin T was normal. The BNP, C-reactive protein and d-dimer were all increased.

The extremely low pO2 concerned the doctor but he did not feel Jun warranted a bed in the ICU at this time. Jun was transferred to the intermediate ICU instead. Linda was sent home. This would be the first time in their fifty-four years of marriage they would be separated.

Upon arrival in the intermediate unity, Jun's vital signs were retaken and were stable. Blood cultures were also done. Samples were taken to confirm the Coronavirus. He was begun on IV fluids (D5/W) at 75 cc/hour. The oxygen was changed to a 40% Venti mask. Strict isolation precautions were enforced. He was begun on IV Remdesivir as well as cefepime and azithromycin as well as Lovenox. The ABGs were repeated. The pO2 was now 56 while his O2 saturation was only 86%. The EKG monitor showed that his heart rate had increased to 132.

The oxygen was increased to a high flow 100% mask and Jun was transferred to the ICU. He was seen at once by the Intensivist who, after discussion by telephone with Linda, intubated Jun. Jun was placed on 100% O2, Assist Control of 16 and a TV of 400 ccs (estimated 6 cc/kg X 70 kg) and 5 cm of PEEP. He was paralyzed and heavily sedated. A Swan-Ganz catheter was placed. The wedge pressure was 22 cm. Normal is less than 18. The chest radiograph was repeated. The ET tube was in good position as was the Swan Ganz catheter. There was no pneumothorax, but the pulmonary infiltrates were much worse. The doctor ordered an echocardiogram which showed that both the left and right ventricle were not contracting normally. They were hypokinetic. Later that day a feeding tube was placed.

The patient's oxygenation improved significantly following the institution of mechanical ventilation. The pO2 increased to 106. But over the next twenty-four hours, the O2 saturation fell. The patient was then transferred to a roto prone positioning bed and placed in the prone position. He was continued on Assist control volume ventilation. Almost immediately Jun's oxygenation improved. The intensivist decided to keep Jun in the prone position 20 hours a day and in the supine position for 4 hours a day.

The next day the ABGs were better. The pO2 was 110, the pCO2 was 48, the pH was 7.32 and the HCO3 was 24. The CXR, however, was much worse. The doctor called Linda and told her that he felt that Jun had myocarditis in addition to his viral pneumonia and that the outlook was poor. He discussed with her what should and should not be done if the situation worsened. He touched on the use of ECMO as well as a trial of dexamethasone, a potent steroid, which showed some success in some patients. Linda agreed to the trial of dexamethasone but did not want the ECMO. Nor did she believe that Jun wanted to have CPR if his heart stopped.

The doctor stopped the azithromycin because of the risk of cardiac arrhythmias in a patient with myocarditis and began a course of high dose dexamethasone. He continued the Remdesivir. The blood tests that day showed a rise in the creatinine, a kidney test, indicating the kidneys were failing.

Over the next five days, Jun's cardiopulmonary condition waxed and waned. However, the renal function continued to deteriorate. The doctor advised Linda that dialysis was needed. Linda said absolutely not. There would be no dialysis and there would be no CPR.

Jun died two days later.

Background for the presentations

The three cases present two contrasting facets of ARDS. In the first case, the cause of ARDS is septic shock which directly affects the capillary endothelium. While the patient's pulmonary status was stable the patient unfortunately died of renal failure and a cardiac arrest due to the sepsis. In the second and third cases, the patients develop ARDS due to infection. In the second case it is due to the disruption of the alveolar type one cells by the influenza virus. In the third case, the Coronavirus caused not only a viral pneumonia, but also a myocarditis with subsequent heart and renal failure.

Important points

1. ARDS is a syndrome caused by diseases which either interfere with the capillary endothelium of the lung or with the type 1 alveolar cells. Thus, it can be caused by either indirect or direct lung injury.
2. In order to diagnosis ARDS there must be an injury or disease entity which is known to cause the syndrome and the patient must have both hypoxemia and interstitial changes on the chest radiograph or CAT scan of the chest.
3. There is no specific treatment for ARDS. The main goal is managing the patient's hypoxemia and treating the underlying cause of the illness.
4. "Lung protective" ventilator settings are paramount. The tidal volume should be limited to 6 cc/Kg body weight and the peak pressure should be less than 30 cm. Sedation may be needed when low lung volume ventilation is used. In addition, at times, the patient may need to be paralyzed when sedation alone is not enough.
5. Both oxygen and pulmonary volutrauma due to shear injury to the alveolar wall can cause ARDS.

6. The patient may have a relatively normal PaO2 but have a markedly abnormal A-a O2 gradient. Always measure the A-a O2 gradient.
7. The treatment of ARDS usually involves a multidisciplinary approach as in the first case.

Discussion

The fluid balance between the capillaries, the interstitial spaces, and the alveoli is dynamic and complex. There are pressures pushing fluid into and out of the capillaries. The capillary and alveolar lining cells are semi-permeable, and their permeability can change. The dynamic forces exerted also changes as blood flows from the arterial side to the venous side of the capillary. In addition, the amount of surfactant in the alveoli directly affects the alveolar surface tension. A high surface tension, due to decreased production of surfactant, will tend to draw fluid into the alveolus.

Starling's law relates the hydrostatic pressure in the capillary, the hydrostatic pressure in the interstitial tissue, the osmotic pressure in the capillary, and the osmotic pressure in the interstitial tissue, as well as the permeability and the reflection coefficient of the capillary barrier, which is defined as the permeability of the capillary membrane to proteins.

Q = K times {(P cap minus P int) − RC times (P osm cap minus P osm int)}

Q is the net movement of fluid out of or into the capillary, K is the liquid conductance or permeability, P cap is the hydrostatic pressure in the capillary, P int is the hydrostatic pressure in the interstitial tissue, RC is the reflection coefficient which is a separate measure of the permeability limited to just proteins and ranges from 0 (completely permeable) to 1 (completely impermeable), P osm cap is the osmotic pressure in the capillary, and P osm int is the osmotic pressure in the interstitial tissue.

On the arterial side, the P cap is much higher than the P int and the difference exceeds the gradient between the osmolarity pressures of the capillary and interstitial tissues. Thus, fluid tends to move out of the capillary into the interstitial tissue. As blood flows through the capillary, the capillary pressure falls and the capillary osmotic pressure rises. Because of these changes at some point the flow is reversed. Fluid flows from the interstitial tissue back into the capillary. If there is more fluid leaving the capillary than returning, the lymph channels in the interstitial tissue carry the fluid off and return it to the blood via the thoracic duct. The lymph channels and the interstitial osmotic pressure and interstitial hydrostatic gradient work to keep the alveoli dry as does the surfactant which lowers the surface pressure in the alveoli.

In a patient with pulmonary venous hypertension from congestive heart failure the flow of fluid returning to the capillary on the venous side is reduced because of the higher pulmonary venous pressure and more fluid pours into the interstitium to be carried off by the lymphatics.

In contrast, patients with non-cardiogenic pulmonary edema (ARDS) have a different and much more substantial problem. In a patient with ARDS, the capillary permeability is increased. Not only do small molecules like sugar leak into the interstitium with the fluid flux, but large proteins do as well. When proteins leak from the capillary into the interstitium, the capillary osmotic pressure is decreased and the interstitial osmotic pressure is increased thus aggravating the flow of fluid out of the capillaries. The fluid floods the interstitium overwhelming the lymphatics. In addition, the type 1 alveolar cells are damaged making the interstitial-alveolar membrane still more permeable. Because the type 2 alveolar cells function is impaired there is decreased surfactant. The leaky alveolar membrane and the decreased surfactant result in fluid flooding the alveoli.

Severe ventilation/perfusion inequality characterized predominantly as "shunting," is the consequence of the capillary flow being maintained through flooded and atelectatic alveoli. This results in hypoxemia. The hypoxemia causes bronchoconstriction and inflammation which worsens the condition.

Thus, ARDS is the final common pathway caused by "inflammation" resulting in increased capillary and alveolar permeability causing the alveoli to become filled with a proteinaceous fluid. The basis of the problem can either be direct, due to alveolar damage, or indirect, due to damage to the capillary endothelial cells.

Direct injury is most often due to pneumonia (40% of patients with ARDS), especially viral pneumonias such as influenza. RSV, or covid. But aspiration of gastric contents, smoke inhalation, steam inhalation and drowning are also culprits. The most common cause of indirect injury is sepsis (32% of patients with ARDS) but fat emboli, transfusions reactions, and massive transfusions (more than 15 units), heroin, aspirin, pancreatitis, chest wall trauma such as a lung contusion, and amniotic fluid embolism can also cause indirect injury. Whether the injury is direct or indirect, inflammation of the alveolar-capillary junction occurs resulting in increased capillary-alveolar permeability.

Over the years since the syndrome was described in the late 1960's and early 1970's, the definition of ARDS has been fine-tuned. The most recent definition is the Berlin Definition of 2012. It states that ARDS is a syndrome characterized by four facets:

1. History of an illness or injury or aggravation of an illness or injury, which is a known cause of ARDS, occurring in the week before the development of hypoxemia.
2. Significant interstitial changes on the chest radiograph.
3. Significant hypoxemia.
4. No evidence of the changes being due solely to cardiogenic pulmonary edema, although the patient may have both cardiogenic pulmonary edema and non-cardiogenic pulmonary edema together.

The syndrome is then divided into three groups based on the ratio between the PaO2 and fiO2:

PaO2/fiO2	severity
200-300	mild
100-200	moderate
<100	severe

There are about 190,000 cases of ARDS a year in the United States. Nearly half of the patients will die. Between 10 and 15% of patients admitted to the ICU have ARDS and about 23% of ventilated patients have ARDS. On the other hand, 80% of patients with ARDS require a ventilator. The incidence of the syndrome increases dramatically with age, but the incidence appears to have decreased overall in the last two decades.

The typical patient develops shortness of breath about 24 to 72 hours after the initiating injury or illness. Examination of the patient shows tachypnea and tachycardia and may show fine inspiratory crackles over the lower lung fields. Over the next few hours, the chest radiograph begins to show patchy interstitial infiltrations which progress in severity. Confusion may be present along with cyanosis and respiratory distress. The laboratory findings reflect the underlying pathology.

The pathologic changes of the lung follow a similar pattern. Initially there is an *exudative phase* characterized by the presence of fluid-filled alveoli with hyaline membranes which are composed of fibrin, cellular debris, and proteins. This is followed by a *proliferative phase* in a few days characterized by hyperplasia of the type 2 alveolocytes, as well as the presence of abundant inflammatory cells and fibroblasts. After another week or two the *fibrotic phase* ensues, characterized by the fibroblasts laying down fibrin or scar tissue resulting in diffuse pulmonary fibrosis.

Clinically, cardiogenic heart failure must be distinguished from ARDS or non-cardiogenic pulmonary edema. A BNP (brain naturetic protein) can be helpful but only if it is normal. If the BNP is less than 100, cardiogenic pulmonary edema is very unlikely. If the BNP is elevated, the illness could be either cardiogenic or non-cardiogenic pulmonary edema and a right heart catheterization may be needed to decide which of the two it is. Measuring the left ventricular end diastolic pressure is, of course, most helpful. A value less than 18 mg hg makes cardiogenic pulmonary edema very unlikely.

Once the diagnosis is established treatment is directed mainly at the initiating event. For example, if the primary cause was sepsis, then antibiotics are necessary. Treatment of ARDS is mainly supportive. There must be meticulous attention to fluid balance. There is an increased risk of thrombophlebitis and pulmonary embolism. In fact, some patients have *disseminated intravascular coagulation* and may develop thromboses in the pulmonary arterioles. Thus, either low molecular weight heparin or intermittent pneumatic compressive stockings should be employed. In addition, gastric ulcers due to stress are quite common. For this reason, the patient should be treated with a proton pump inhibitor such as Protonix. Sedation may be needed, especially if the patient is treated with pressure-controlled ventilation, but sedation should be kept to a minimum. In fact, patients who are more alert do better than patients who are sedated. A more controversial topic is the use of neuromuscular blockade in order to paralyze the patient while he or she is being ventilated. One study several years ago showed that patients treated with neuromuscular blockade had more ventilator-free days in the first one to three months and were less likely to have barotrauma. Overall, it appears that only those patients with severe ARDS will benefit from neuromuscular blockade. In addition, neuromuscular blockade requires that the patient be completely sedated and that may result in prolonged muscular weakness.

Nutritional support is also important. Patients with ARDS have a higher energy expenditure and additional nutritional support is needed. This should be given via the gastrointestinal tract where possible. But overfeeding needs to be avoided as well, as it can raise glucose to unacceptable levels.

Care must be taken to prevent nosocomial infections, especially pulmonary infections, in the patient with ARDS. Hand washing between patients, elevating the head of the patient's bed and strict standard guidelines for the ventilated patient must be strenuously adhered to.

As of this moment there is no evidence that glucocorticoids will prevent ARDS or treat ARDS in general. They should only be used if the underlying disease or illness which caused the ARDS will benefit from steroid therapy, although the Society of Critical Care Medicine recently suggested that the early use of steroids may be beneficial in patients with moderate to severe ARDS unresponsive to standard care. In addition, the use of intravenous dexamethasone for treating patients with severe covid is well accepted.

Fluid management should err on the conservative side. A central venous catheter should be used to monitor the central venous pressure which should be kept at less than 4 cm. While the ARDS patient is suffering from the effects of increased capillary permeability, anything which increases the capillary interstitial pressure will increase the fluid flux out of the capillary and into the interstitium. Maintaining the patient in a "dry state" without, of course, impairing renal function or causing low blood pressure should be done.

Another ancillary technique that has been shown to be efficacious in patients with ARDS is the use of prone positioning during ventilation. Prone positioning results in better distribution of ventilation and ventilation/perfusion matching. It is imperative that the hospital staff be well-trained in executing the change from supine to prone and prone to supine positions to prevent complications.

Hypoxemia is the primary problem faced by patients with ARDS. The goal is to keep the paO2 at 60 or more. Because the underlying problem in these patients is "shunting," low flow oxygen just is not going to be enough. High flow nasal oxygen can be tried and may be helpful in some patients. If the patient can't maintain a paO2 greater than 60 on a 60% high flow Venti mask, then either non-invasive ventilation (NIV) or invasive ventilation with an endotracheal tube need to be done. If the patient has mild ARDS and a condition which is likely to resolve in 1 to 3 days such as fat embolism syndrome, a transfusion reaction, or a viral pneumonia, non-invasive ventilation is a good choice. Again, the goal is to maintain the paO2 at more than 60. NIV can be used with higher amounts of oxygen and PEEP up to 10-15 cm.

One study alluded to above showed that early neuromuscular blockade with the use of sedation improved mortality in patients with severe ARDS. However, a recent study in the NEJM failed to confirm this finding.[2] An accompanying editorial by Arthur Slutsky and Jesus Villar suggested the difference between the two studies may have been due to the presence of "dyssynchrony reverse

---

[2] The National Heart, Lung, and Blood Institute PETAL Clinical Trial Network; Early Neuromuscular Blockade in the Acute Respiratory Distress Syndrome; NEJM, 2019, 380: 1997-2008

triggering" in the control subjects of the earlier trial who were heavily sedated. In this condition, the ventilator triggered the patient to take a spontaneous breath resulting in breath stacking, higher PEEP, and more volutrauma. Thus, the control patients were at a disadvantage compared to the paralyzed and sedated experimental patients. Based on the most recent study, at the present time, routine paralysis, and sedation of patients with ARDS is not advised.

There is a definite risk to oxygen given at more than 50%. Damage to the lungs occurs within just a few hours in animal studies. ARDSNET recommendations should be strictly adhered to.

If the patient needs to be placed on a ventilator, then care must be taken to prevent complications from intubation and the use of the ventilator. In the immediate period before and after intubation the patient should be placed on 90-95% oxygen. The advantages to using invasive ventilation include the ability to deliver higher amounts of oxygen and PEEP as well as to have more control of the patient's ventilation allowing the use of sedation and neuromuscular blockade if needed.

In general, there are two modes of ventilator therapy. Either pressure or volume can be used to limit the amount of ventilation the patient receives. In the pressure mode, the ventilator delivers gas to the patient until the set pressure is reached. In the volume mode, the ventilator delivers gas to the patient until the set volume is reached. Secondary settings can override the primary settings. For example, in the volume control mode, a maximum pressure can also be set. The tidal breath may be set to deliver 600 cc but if the patient exceeds a preset pressure the machine will stop delivering gas to the patient so as not to exceed that pressure.

There are two forms of pressure limited ventilation: pressure support ventilation (PSV) and pressure-controlled ventilation (PCV). With PSV the patient takes a breath which is sensed by the ventilator which then delivers gas at a preset positive pressure to the airways. When the patient's airflow slows, the positive pressure is stopped. Its main advantage is that it is certain that the patient will receive comfortable and well-tolerated ventilatory assistance. Its main drawback is that the volume of each breath will be quite variable and unpredictable. In the PCV mode, on the other hand, the ventilator initiates the breath, and the duration of inspiration and expiration are set by the physician. This mode of ventilation is the least patient friendly and sedation is generally required. It is used most often in patients with severe, refractory ARDS.

There are three forms of volume limited ventilation. The first is rarely used today and is controlled volume ventilation in which the ventilator delivers a gas at a respiratory rate, volume and O2 concentration determined by the physician. Much more commonly, the "assist control" mode is used. In this mode the ventilator senses when the patient starts a breath and then delivers the controlled volume of gas to the patient. There is a back-up rate to ensure that the patient gets a set number of breaths every minute. The last type of volume limited ventilation is "synchronized intermittent mandatory ventilation" or SIMV. In this setting the patient is allowed to breathe normally while the machine assists the patient by providing a preset lung volume a preset number of times a minute.

Both pressure and volume limited ventilators have secondary settings to allow for total control or to allow for patient triggered control. The most commonly used mode of ventilation today is "assist controlled volume ventilation." In this mode, when the patient initiates a breath, the ventilator will deliver a set volume of gas to the patient so long as it does not result in the pressure exceeding a preset amount.

In the past the ventilator would be set to deliver 10 cc of gas per kilogram of body weight. More and more evidence has accumulated in recent years showing that these large tidal volumes result in the shearing of the alveolar walls, causing inflammation and the development of ARDS. As a response to this, low tidal volume ventilation (LTVV) or "lung protective ventilation" has been introduced. LTVV has been shown in patients with ARDS to reduce mortality when compared with higher volume ventilation. In fact, just changing the LTVV from 6 cc/kg to 7 cc/kg resulted in a 23% increase in ICU mortality. The main drawback to LTVV is the development of respiratory acidosis, which is generally mild, but may be severe. In addition, there is more asynchrony between the patient and the ventilator resulting in the need for additional sedation, at least initially. Breath-stacking has been shown to be more frequent, even in the sedated patient. If that occurs then the tidal volume should be increased slightly, from 6 cc/kg to 7 cc/kg, as long as the plateau pressure is less than 30 cm.

Protocols should be used to determine initial ventilator settings based on predicted body weight as well as volume and respiratory rate adjustments during the time the patient is on the ventilator. The plateau pressure must be acidulously measured. The goal is for the ventilator to deliver the patient's entire minute ventilation.

PEEP can be adjusted to improve alveolar recruitment so long as the plateau pressure remains under thirty cm. Extremely high PEEP has not been shown to improve the outcome of patients with ARDS. Moreover, PEEP has never been shown to prevent ARDS from developing.

If the patient has severe ARDS and remains refractory to conventional therapy extracorporeal membrane oxygenation (ECMO) is certainly a realistic option. The survival rate in those patients with a PaO2/fiO2 of less than 100 has improved with ECMO. In essence the patient's circulation is diverted from the right atrium into a machine which both oxygenates the blood and removes carbon dioxide. Then the blood is returned to the patient via the right atrium. ECMO is essentially "lung replacement therapy." ECMO may even serve as a bridge to a lung transplant.

During the use of ECMO the patient must be anticoagulated with low molecular weight heparin or a direct thrombin inhibitor. Platelets are damaged during ECMO, and the platelet level must be followed closely. Platelet transfusions can be given as needed. Of importance, the ventilator settings must be reduced, especially the plateau pressure, which should be set at less than 20 cm and the fiO2 at less than 0.5. Reducing the plateau pressure will improve cardiac output and reducing the fiO2 will decrease further risk of ARDS.

The main risks of ECMO are bleeding, thromboembolism, and neurologic damage. Bleeding is a risk because the patient has both a low platelet count and is on blood thinners. Thrombosis can occur in the extracorporeal circuit. Neurologic damage occurs in about 10% of patients treated with ECMO.

Over the last three decades the incidence of ARDS has decreased and the science behind the treatment of the disorder has improved significantly. Nevertheless, ARDS is still a major killer in the ICU, and this demands that patient care be continuously monitored and improved.

Suggestions for minor papers

1. What is sepsis?
2. What is "lung protective ventilation?"
3. What are the complications of non-invasive ventilation?
4. What are the consequences of invasive ventilation?
5. What are the ARDSNET recommendations?
6. How is using the prone position helpful?
7. What is the "roto prone bed" and how does it help oxygenation?
8. Compare pressure-controlled versus volume-controlled ventilation.
9. Discuss "barotrauma" and "volutrauma."

Peter A. Petroff, MD

Seminars in Respiratory Disease

Six

Congestive Heart Failure

Heart disease is the number one killer in the United States. 6,000,000 Americans have heart failure and more than 600,000 die of heart disease yearly. The five-year mortality of people with heart disease is 42%. In other words, almost half of patients with heart disease die within five years. The life expectancy is half that of an untreated patient with the HIV virus. Diseases of the coronary arteries, the blood supply to the heart, account for more than half the deaths. The main risk factors for developing heart disease are hypertension, diabetes, high cholesterol and smoking but obesity, physical inactivity, and excessive alcohol are also contributing factors.

The end stage of heart disease could be a heart attack, a fatal heart arrhythmia or congestive heart failure. Heart failure occurs when the heart cannot pump enough blood and oxygen to support the other organs in your body.

There are two types of heart failure. Systolic heart failure is due to a weak heart. The heart muscle is damaged so that the heart is unable to pump effectively. It is most often due to coronary artery disease but can also be due to inflammation of the heart muscle which is called a "cardiomyopathy." Diastolic heart failure is due to a very hypertrophied and stiff left ventricle. It is most often due to hypertension or to an aortic valve whose opening has become narrowed by scarring. While the symptoms of both types of heart failure are similar, their therapies differ as well as their prognoses.

The treatment of heart failure includes medicines to reduce the amount of work the heart must perform. These are called "afterload reducers" and include both the angiotensin converting enzyme inhibitors and the angiotensin receptor blockers. B adrenergic agents are used to decrease how strongly the heart contracts and thus reduce the heart's need for oxygen. Diuretics or "water pills" are used to reduce the size of the heart when it is in diastole thus increasing how effectively the heart can contract. In addition, MRA's or mineral cortical receptor antagonists, and three new types of medications, ARNI's, SGLT2 (**S**erum **Gl**ucose Co-**T**ransmitters 2) inhibitors, and Guanyl cyclase stimulants, are becoming part of the standard care.

Peter A. Petroff, MD

Case Studies

1

Max is an 82-year-old man who has poorly controlled Type 2 Diabetes and a long history of hypertension. He has been short of breath for a few months. However, the night before admission to the hospital he was forced to sleep sitting in a chair. He could not lie down without becoming extremely short of breath.

Max has been diabetic for more than twenty years. His most recent hemoglobin A1C was 8.5. The normal value is less than 5.7. He is currently taking Metformin and insulin to treat his diabetes. He has been hypertensive for ten years and is taking Vasotec, Hydrochlorothiazide, and a baby aspirin. He also takes Plavix, a blood thinner, and Crestor, a medication to lower cholesterol. His past history is significant in that he had two heart attacks in the past. The first one was five years ago and was quite severe. He had pressure in his chest that lasted six hours before he went to the emergency room. He was found to have a 95% blockage of his left anterior descending coronary artery. The cardiologist did an emergency balloon angioplasty, and placed a stent Despite the medical interventions, part of the wall of his left ventricle was damaged. The following year he had another heart attack which, while not as severe, resulted in still more damage to his heart. After the second heart attack, his left ventricular ejection fraction was about 40% of predicted as measured by echocardiogram. The normal value is more than 55%.

After his second heart attack he quit smoking. He had smoked about a pack a day for more than 45 years. After quitting smoking, he gained weight, going from 175 lbs. to more than 230 lbs. About a year ago he became much more sedentary. All he did all day was sit at home watching the television. Once a day he would take his dog for a short walk. If he walked more than two blocks, he became short of breath. He also noted that his feet were swelling especially in late afternoon. About a month ago the shortness of breath began getting worse. He could no longer walk his dog. He could not fit in his shoes. He states he did not have any chest pain or pressure in his chest. "I was just shorter of breath, doc." Then last night, the breathing became unbearable.

His additional past history is significant. He drinks about two Martinis a day, sometimes more. He has not had any surgery or other medical admissions. He states he takes his medicines regularly and has no drug allergies. His mother died at sixty-one from a heart attack. His father died of a stroke at fifty-five.

His physical exam revealed him to be a moderately obese male who was short of breath even at rest. His lips were slightly cyanotic. He had audible wheezing.

The patient removed his shirt and lay on the examining table with the head of the table at 30 degrees. Examination of his lungs showed fine inspiratory crackles in both lung bases with scattered expiratory wheezes which cleared somewhat with coughing. Examination of the heart showed moderate neck vein distention. The heart was enlarged to percussion. The S1 (first heart sound) was decreased and there was an S3 gallop. The abdomen showed that the liver was enlarged to percussion. There was 2 + pitting edema below the knees.

The patient was admitted to the ICU. On arrival his blood pressure was 155/96, his pulse was 142 and his respiratory rate was 18. He was 5' 8" tall and he weighed 236 lbs.

The doctor ordered a chest radiograph, EKG, CBC, Chemistry profile, a BNP, cardiac enzymes, troponin levels, urinalysis and ABGs. He began Max on oxygen at 2 l/min using a nasal cannula. He also ordered the patient be given 40 mg of Lasix intravenously.

The chest radiograph showed bibasilar interstitial changes with small Kerley B lines bilaterally. The heart was markedly enlarged with left ventricular predominance. The EKG showed a regular rhythm with evidence of an old anterolateral myocardial infarct. The CBC was normal. The chemistry profile showed that the sugar was quite high at 287 while the kidney function was slightly impaired. The creatinine was 1.6. (Normal value is less than 1.2) The BNP or brain naturetic protein *was over a thousand. The Cardiac Troponin studies were normal. The urinalysis showed 2+ protein. The blood gases on oxygen showed a pH of 7.45, a pO2 of 75, a pCO2 of 46 and a HCO3 of 30.*

Over the next hour the patient diuresed more than a liter and a half of clear urine and felt much better.

The doctor then ordered an echocardiogram which showed his left ventricular function had worsened. He now had a markedly dilated left ventricle with an ejection fraction of only 28%. He had stage four heart disease. The doctor said he had "HFrEF."

The patient was begun on a beta blocker (Toprol) in addition to his Vasotec. He was changed from hydrochlorothiazide which he took at home to furosemide (Lasix). The doctor prescribed Spironolactone, an aldosterone antagonist, to his regimen.

The following morning Max felt "better than I've felt in more than a year." The doctor repeated the EKG and troponin studies. There was nothing to suggest another heart attack. Max demanded that he be allowed to go home. He promised to come to the office the next morning.

The next day, the doctor was late getting to his office, so he came in by the front door rather than the staff entrance. As he walked through the waiting room, he saw Max sitting in a comfortable chair sound asleep. The doctor looked closely; Max was not breathing. Then, as if on signal, Max began to try to breathe. His stomach and chest fought each other as he struggled for a breath; finally, Max took a breath. He looked up then to the right turning his body a little. In just a few seconds, he had drifted off again. His head fell onto his chin and his breathing stopped. The doctor shook him. Max looked up, "Hi doc!" The doctor shook his head, "Follow me."

The two walked into the office together. The nurse took Max's vital signs, and the doctor began to speak. He told Max he had end-stage heart disease, and he wanted Max to get a sleep study and have an implantable cardiac defibrillator placed in his heart. Max surprisingly agreed to both requests.

2.

Allison is a 55-year-old woman who presents to the emergency room extremely short of breath. On the patient's arrival in the ER, the triage nurse begins her on oxygen and notifies the doctor who tells her to get an EKG, chest radiograph, ABGs and CBC "stat."

As soon as the doctor is free, he hurries to see Allison. She states that she was well until a year ago when she began having shortness of breath. At first it was mild and intermittent. Sometimes she could hear wheezes. She notes that she had asthma as a child. She went to her doctor who diagnosed her with asthma and began her on an Albuterol spray. When it did not help, he added an inhaled steroid. She used the medications regularly and cut back on her activities and was able to get by. About a month ago she had an episode of severe crushing chest pain which brought her to her knees. "It seemed to come out of the blue. I was late and I was rushing. But the pain stopped me in my tracks." She points to her chest with a closed fist. She went back to the doctor who gave her Protonix for acid reflux and scheduled her for some tests.

Allison states that the tests are scheduled to be done in a week but today she was so short of breath she couldn't even dress. Worse still, the pain came back again. Instead of calling her doctor, she called an ambulance and was brought to the hospital emergency room.

Allison does not smoke or drink. She takes only her Albuterol and steroid spray. She has no allergies. She has not had any surgery. She has never been hospitalized. Her parents died when she was quite young. She does not know the cause of their deaths. She has no history of heart disease, but she recalls that when she tried out for sports in high school the doctor found a murmur. He did an EKG and told her not to worry about it.

The nurse took her vital signs. Her height was 5' 3". Her weight was 98 lbs. Her BP was 108/68 and her pulse was 138. The nurse noted that the pulse was quite weak and difficult to feel. She was breathing fast.

Examination of her head and neck was unremarkable save mildly cyanotic lips and a noticeably weak carotid pulse. Her lungs showed diffuse crackles over all lung fields. Examination of her heart showed a grade 3 systolic murmur over the entire heart but especially at the 2nd right interspace. The murmur began after the first heart sound and ended before the second. It was soft than got loud and then soft again. The doctor said, "crescendo-decrescendo." Examination of her abdomen showed the liver was slightly enlarged. There was no edema.

The chest x-ray showed diffuse interstitial changes in a "butterfly" pattern. The heart was normal in size. The blood count was normal. The EKG showed left ventricular enlargement. The blood gases showed a pO2 of 54, a pCO2 of 35, a pH of 7.48 and an HCO3 of 24.

The doctor told the lab to do a BNP "stat." He also ordered an immediate echocardiogram. He began the patient on oxygen and gave her morphine sulfate to relax her as well as a dose of furosemide (Lasix).

decreased and there was an S3 gallop. The abdomen showed that the liver was enlarged to percussion. There was 2 + pitting edema below the knees.

The patient was admitted to the ICU. On arrival his blood pressure was 155/96, his pulse was 142 and his respiratory rate was 18. He was 5' 8" tall and he weighed 236 lbs.

The doctor ordered a chest radiograph, EKG, CBC, Chemistry profile, a BNP, cardiac enzymes, troponin levels, urinalysis and ABGs. He began Max on oxygen at 2 l/min using a nasal cannula. He also ordered the patient be given 40 mg of Lasix intravenously.

The chest radiograph showed bibasilar interstitial changes with small Kerley B lines bilaterally. The heart was markedly enlarged with left ventricular predominance. The EKG showed a regular rhythm with evidence of an old anterolateral myocardial infarct. The CBC was normal. The chemistry profile showed that the sugar was quite high at 287 while the kidney function was slightly impaired. The creatinine was 1.6. (Normal value is less than 1.2) The BNP or brain naturetic protein *was over a thousand. The Cardiac Troponin studies were normal. The urinalysis showed 2+ protein. The blood gases on oxygen showed a pH of 7.45, a pO2 of 75, a pCO2 of 46 and a HCO3 of 30.*

Over the next hour the patient diuresed more than a liter and a half of clear urine and felt much better.

The doctor then ordered an echocardiogram which showed his left ventricular function had worsened. He now had a markedly dilated left ventricle with an ejection fraction of only 28%. He had stage four heart disease. The doctor said he had "HFrEF."

The patient was begun on a beta blocker (Toprol) in addition to his Vasotec. He was changed from hydrochlorothiazide which he took at home to furosemide (Lasix). The doctor prescribed Spironolactone, an aldosterone antagonist, to his regimen.

The following morning Max felt "better than I've felt in more than a year." The doctor repeated the EKG and troponin studies. There was nothing to suggest another heart attack. Max demanded that he be allowed to go home. He promised to come to the office the next morning.

The next day, the doctor was late getting to his office, so he came in by the front door rather than the staff entrance. As he walked through the waiting room, he saw Max sitting in a comfortable chair sound asleep. The doctor looked closely; Max was not breathing. Then, as if on signal, Max began to try to breathe. His stomach and chest fought each other as he struggled for a breath; finally, Max took a breath. He looked up then to the right turning his body a little. In just a few seconds, he had drifted off again. His head fell onto his chin and his breathing stopped. The doctor shook him. Max looked up, "Hi doc!" The doctor shook his head, "Follow me."

The two walked into the office together. The nurse took Max's vital signs, and the doctor began to speak. He told Max he had end-stage heart disease, and he wanted Max to get a sleep study and have an implantable cardiac defibrillator placed in his heart. Max surprisingly agreed to both requests.

2.

Allison is a 55-year-old woman who presents to the emergency room extremely short of breath. On the patient's arrival in the ER, the triage nurse begins her on oxygen and notifies the doctor who tells her to get an EKG, chest radiograph, ABGs and CBC "stat."

As soon as the doctor is free, he hurries to see Allison. She states that she was well until a year ago when she began having shortness of breath. At first it was mild and intermittent. Sometimes she could hear wheezes. She notes that she had asthma as a child. She went to her doctor who diagnosed her with asthma and began her on an Albuterol spray. When it did not help, he added an inhaled steroid. She used the medications regularly and cut back on her activities and was able to get by. About a month ago she had an episode of severe crushing chest pain which brought her to her knees. "It seemed to come out of the blue. I was late and I was rushing. But the pain stopped me in my tracks." She points to her chest with a closed fist. She went back to the doctor who gave her Protonix for acid reflux and scheduled her for some tests.

Allison states that the tests are scheduled to be done in a week but today she was so short of breath she couldn't even dress. Worse still, the pain came back again. Instead of calling her doctor, she called an ambulance and was brought to the hospital emergency room.

Allison does not smoke or drink. She takes only her Albuterol and steroid spray. She has no allergies. She has not had any surgery. She has never been hospitalized. Her parents died when she was quite young. She does not know the cause of their deaths. She has no history of heart disease, but she recalls that when she tried out for sports in high school the doctor found a murmur. He did an EKG and told her not to worry about it.

The nurse took her vital signs. Her height was 5' 3". Her weight was 98 lbs. Her BP was 108/68 and her pulse was 138. The nurse noted that the pulse was quite weak and difficult to feel. She was breathing fast.

Examination of her head and neck was unremarkable save mildly cyanotic lips and a noticeably weak carotid pulse. Her lungs showed diffuse crackles over all lung fields. Examination of her heart showed a grade 3 systolic murmur over the entire heart but especially at the 2nd right interspace. The murmur began after the first heart sound and ended before the second. It was soft than got loud and then soft again. The doctor said, "crescendo-decrescendo." Examination of her abdomen showed the liver was slightly enlarged. There was no edema.

The chest x-ray showed diffuse interstitial changes in a "butterfly" pattern. The heart was normal in size. The blood count was normal. The EKG showed left ventricular enlargement. The blood gases showed a pO2 of 54, a pCO2 of 35, a pH of 7.48 and an HCO3 of 24.

The doctor told the lab to do a BNP "stat." He also ordered an immediate echocardiogram. He began the patient on oxygen and gave her morphine sulfate to relax her as well as a dose of furosemide (Lasix).

The BNP was extremely elevated consistent with congestive heart failure. The echocardiogram showed marked thickening of the walls of the left ventricle. The aortic valve was calcified and the cross-sectional area of the aortic valve opening between the left ventricle and the aorta was markedly narrowed. The echocardiogram technician told her the opening appeared "critically narrowed."

The doctor concluded she had critical aortic valve stenosis causing diastolic heart failure. He realized at once that diuretics and afterload reducers were going to be ineffective. He discussed his findings with her. He suggested that heart surgery was needed immediately.

After the cardiovascular surgeon examined the patient, he felt the situation was serious, if not critical. He recommended a trans-catheter aortic valve replacement (TAVR) and scheduled it for the following morning

The following morning the procedure was carried out. Within an hour after the procedure Allison noted that her breathing was much better. Because the risk of atrial fibrillation is quite high after the TAVR, she was begun on anticoagulation.

She continued to improve and was discharged from the hospital two days later on only the blood thinner. She was no longer short of breath. At the time of discharge her blood pressure was 124/86, her pulse was 84. Her O2 saturation was 96%. She was scheduled to see the surgeon in one month.

3.

Beth D. is a 28-year-old woman who was brought to the emergency room by ambulance. She is extremely short of breath. She speaks in short sentences. She is sallow and appears wasted, but she has marked pedal edema as well as abdominal distention. The nurse in the ER places her on oxygen and applies the electrodes needed for the cardiac monitor. The emergency medical technician tells the nurse that they were called by the patient's husband. The husband refused to give any history and did not accompany the patient to the hospital.

The doctor arrives in a few minutes. He orders a chest radiograph and ABGs as well as a CBC, chemistry profile, Troponin T, BNP, and urinalysis. He asks the nurse to insert a foley catheter and do an EKG.

As the nurse does the EKG, the doctor speaks to Beth. She states she has been short of breath for months. "At least six or eight months." She has had chest pain. "The pain is right here, and it goes here." She draws a line on her chest with her right hand running from just left of the lower sternum up to her left shoulder. "It came on anytime." "The only way I got any relief was to sit up and lean forward." "Then it was all the time." She states she couldn't eat. Despite not eating much at all, her weight increased, and her stomach swelled. Her feet swelled as well.

Over the last month, she has become bedridden. "I sit in my sofa and sleep most of the day and night."

She has had a productive cough with green phlegm. She has not been feverish. "But I sweat a lot at night." She has been fatigued for more than a year. "That is when I began to lose weight." She doesn't smoke. "Never liked it, like my hubby does." She does not drink. She doesn't take any medicine, prescribed or otherwise.

Her past history is significant. She grew up in poverty and never finished high school. Her parents died when she was young, and she was lived with her grandmother for a while. Her grandmother died of tuberculosis when Beth was twelve. She then lived with an aunt and then went into foster care till she was eighteen when she married. "He is totally worthless." She has not had any surgery nor been in the hospital for any reason. She has never seen a doctor.

The nurse hands the doctor the EKG: *The EKG shows a sinus rhythm. There are no acute changes, but the ST segments are elevated in all the precordial leads.*

The vital signs are as follows: the B/P is 86/64, the pulse is 128, the height is estimated to be 5 feet, four inches, the weight is 88 lbs.

Her physical exam shows her to have a sallow complexion with sunken cheeks. Her lips are cyanotic. Her neck veins are distended to the angle of her jaw even when the doctor raises the head of the bed to 30 degrees. The examination of her lungs is normal. The heart sounds are barely audible. The first and second heart sounds are normal and there are no murmurs. The doctor examines her chest wall. Her breasts are tiny and free of nodules. Her abdomen is markedly distended and dull to percussion. The doctor tells the nurse, "This is ascites." He could not feel the liver or spleen because of the swelling. She also had 2+ pedal edema. All her pulses were barely palpable.

The x-ray technician arrives as does the laboratory technician. In a quarter hour, the results are ready.

The chest x-ray shows a large heart that look like a big balloon in a little chest. The lungs show fibrocalcific changes in the left upper lobe. There are no signs of congestive heart failure. The chemistry profile is normal as is the Troponin T. The BNP is slightly elevated. The CBC shows a moderate anemia with a hemoglobin of 9.6 (Normal is 12-16). The urinalysis is normal.

The doctor looks at the chest radiograph on the computer terminal in the ER. He turns to the nurse and says, "We need a "stat" cardiac ultrasound."

The cardiac technician arrives in a few minutes. The doctor looks over her shoulder as she carries out the study. He says quietly, "As I expected, a large pericardial effusion. The fluid is causing her to have heart failure." He sits next to Beth, "The heart sits inside a sack. Normally there is a little fluid in the sack, but you have a lot of fluid. You have so much fluid that your heart can't expand normally. That's what's causing your breathing to be so short. We have to remove the fluid immediately." He then discusses the procedure in detail as well as some of the things that could go wrong. Beth appears terrified but after a few seconds she says vehemently, "If I die so what, I can't live like this."

The doctor then calls the radiologist, and the patient is taken to the x-ray department where the radiologist performs a pericardiocentesis. After topical anesthesia, he inserts a tube just below the lowest rib and to the left of midline. The tube is directed up and to the right. As the tube enters the pericardial sack, Beth startles and grabs the side of the table. Thick pussy fluid drains from tube. More than a liter of fluid is removed. As the fluid is removed, Beth relaxes, "I can breathe. I can breathe."

The fluid is sent for several studies including cytology for cancer cells, cultures for tuberculosis and fungi as well as bacteria and a cell count and differential. Beth is then transferred to the ICU on oxygen.

The hospital intensivist reexamines Beth. He also orders sputum for tuberculosis and fungi. He also orders acute viral studies, but he doubts that Beth has a viral pericarditis. He repeats the EKG and Chest radiograph.

The EKG is unchanged. The chest x-ray again shows the scarring at the left upper lobs. The heart no longer appears like a large balloon but there is air in the pericardial space and the pericardium appears thickened.

The doctor also orders a PPD.

Beth does well. Her appetite is definitely better as is her breathing. She diuresed more than 2000 ccs over the next eight hours. By the following morning, her color was better, the cyanosis was gone, the neck veins were no longer "up to her jaws," her abdomen was a little smaller and her legs a little less swollen. Her blood pressure was now 110/72; her pulse was 98. Her oxygen saturation was 98%. The chest x-ray was unchanged. She was transferred to an isolation room in the intermediate ICU. The intensivist asked for an infectious disease and cardiology consult.

The following day, the studies for TB came back positive and she was seen by the infectious disease specialist who began her on four medications for TB including isoniazid, rifampin, ethambutal, and pyrazinamide. The cardiologist ordered a CAT scan of her chest which showed that while the fluid was gone the pericardial sac was thickened. He felt she should have a "pericardial window." After discussion with the patient, a thoracic surgeon was called in. He agreed with the conclusion of the cardiologist but felt the procedure could wait a week or so while the patient was recovering from her acute illness.

Ten days later the surgeon did the pericardial window and a week later the patient was sent home on medicines for tuberculosis.

Background for the Case Presentations

The three cases represent different aspects of congestive heart failure. The first case is a patient with systolic heart failure due to recurrent myocardial infarctions (heart attacks) weakening the left ventricular wall. The second case is a patient with diastolic heart failure due to aortic valvular stenosis or narrowing of the opening (referred to as the orifice) of the aortic outflow tract due to hardening of the leaflets of the aortic valve. Most of the time, aortic stenosis is a result of a congenital bicuspid valve. The third case is entirely different. In this case, the heart muscle is totally normal. The sac that the heart sits in is thickened and the sac is filled with fluid. There is so much fluid that the heart is unable to relax in diastole causing the symptoms and signs of heart failure. Chronic calcific pericarditis is a rare complication of tuberculosis.

Important Points

1. Physiologically heart failure is defined as the inability of the heart to provide adequate oxygen and nutrition for the tissues of the body. Clinically, it is defined as the presence of signs or symptoms of heart failure in the presence of an elevated BNP or evidence of congestion in either the lungs or the systemic circulation or both.
2. In the past heart failure was either systolic heart failure or diastolic heart failure. Currently heart failure is divided into three groups: those with preserved left ventricular ejection fraction (>50 and referred to as HFpEF), those with reduced ejection fraction (< 40 and referred to as HFrEF), and those who have mildly reduced ejection fractions (41-49; referred to as HFmrEF).
3. The signs and symptoms of heart failure are due to both "forward failure" and "backward failure." Forward heart failure results in decreased blood flow to the tissues especially the kidneys and brain. The decreased flow to the kidneys turns on the renin-angiotensin-aldosterone pathway which leads to salt retention. The decreased flow to the carotid bodies and brain activates the sympathetic system causing tachycardia as well as sweating, confusion and other neurological concerns. Backward failure causes the build-up of fluid in the lungs, liver, and feet as well as neck vein distention.
4. In systolic heart failure or HFrEF, the heart is <u>volume overloaded</u>, the left ventricle (or for that matter, the entire heart) is dilated, and the contractility is decreased. Systolic heart failure is most often due to arteriosclerotic heart disease or to mitral valve insufficiency.
5. In diastolic heart failure or HFpEF, the <u>diastolic volume is markedly decreased</u> due to thickening of the wall of the left ventricle. Diastolic heart failure is most often due to hypertension or to aortic valvular stenosis.
6. Systolic and diastolic heart failure can best be evaluated using the echocardiogram. Systolic heart failure will show a dilated left ventricle with a decreased left ventricular ejection fraction (LVEF). Diastolic heart failure will show a thickened left ventricular wall and a normal ejection fraction.
7. Treatment of systolic heart failure involves lowering the afterload, preload and, if necessary, increasing the contractility of the heart. Treatment of diastolic heart failure involves treating the underlying cause (hypertension or aortic stenosis). The prognosis for CHF is poor. The average life expectancy is only five years.
8. One other condition that can rarely result in diastolic heart failure is "restrictive heart failure" due to thickening of the pericardium or the pericardial sac bulging with fluid. In this condition the heart is unable to relax.

Discussion

The Egyptians knew the importance of the heart. For them, it was the seat of good and evil. When a Pharaoh died and was embalmed, all the internal organs were removed and placed in jars outside the body except for the heart which was buried with him. Before the heart was returned to the dead Pharaoh its weight was compared to the weight of an ostrich feather. If the heart weighed less than the feather, the Pharaoh had a good heart and would enjoy the afterlife. If it weighed more than the feather, it was considered to be filled with evil and would be consumed by a god in the guise of a dog. The pharaoh was condemned to a second death and eternal torment. Woe to the Pharaoh with cardiomegaly and congestive heart failure.

The heart is a muscle the size of your fist. It has three layers of muscles: one wraps circumferentially around the heart, one wraps obliquely around the heart, and one wraps around the heart like a spiral. When the muscles contract, they wring out the blood like you wring out the water from a wet towel. The heart, as we all know, has four valves and four chambers, the thinnest of which, the right atrium, has a paper-thin wall, while the thickest, the left ventricle, is more than a centimeter thick. The heart has a low-pressure side, the right atrium and ventricle, and a high- pressure side, the left atrium and ventricle. It has a sophisticated electrical system which allows the atrium to contract and fill the ventricles before they contract. It is innervated by both the parasympathetic and sympathetic nervous systems. It has a blood supply consisting of two main arteries that arise from the aorta just above the takeoff of the aortic valve. The left main coronary artery is short and divides into the anterior descending artery and the circumflex artery. These arteries largely supply the left ventricle. The right main coronary artery supplies the posterior and inferior surface of the heart including the right ventricle.

In one sense we can compare the properties of the heart to the properties of a balloon. The larger we blow up the balloon the more air will be expelled when we release our hold on it. So, the amount of air filling the balloon is the *preload*. If we blow up a balloon with an elastic wall and a balloon with a flimsy wall the one with the elastic wall will expel the air faster. We call that property, how fast the balloon will empty, the *contractility*. Lastly, we can attach a valve to the mouth of the balloon. The tighter we close the valve the slower the air will be expelled. We call the force against which the balloon, and of course the heart must work, the *afterload*.

These three properties, the preload, the contractility, and at the afterload, are the parameters which describe how much blood the heart can pump. The preload is the volume of the heart before it begins to contract. The contractility is the strength of the contraction. The afterload is the mean aortic blood pressure against which the heart must work. The *cardiac output* is the amount of blood expelled in a minute by the heart, while the *stroke volume* is the amount of blood expelled by the heart with each beat.

The Frank-Starling law compares the preload (resting volume of the left ventricle also called the diastolic volume) to the stroke volume (SV); the greater the preload (the more blood in the left ventricle at rest) the greater the stroke volume up to a point. If the heart is stretched too much the stroke volume falls off. The more contractility the heart has the more stroke volume there will be for any given preload. In other words, the curve for the relationship of stroke volume to preload will be higher. B adrenergic agents, thyroid hormone, and the drug digoxin increase the contractility. B blockers decrease the contractility. However, the greater the contractility, the more oxygen the heart requires! In other words, it takes more oxygen to make the heart work harder.

The third relationship we need to consider is that between the stroke volume or cardiac output and the afterload or mean aortic pressure. The greater the afterload the less the cardiac output; in other words, the greater the mean aortic blood pressure the less the cardiac output.

When we discuss the treatment of heart failure, we will see how important these three parameters are. Every treatment we use either lowers the afterload, lowers the preload or raises or lowers the contractility.

Congestive heart failure (CHF) results in the inability of the heart to deliver needed nutrients to the body as a whole. There are two diametrically opposed causes of CHF: systolic heart failure (HFrEF or heart failure with reduced ejection fraction) and diastolic heart failure (HFpEF or heart failure with preserved ejection fraction). Systole is the contraction of the heart. Therefore, heart failure due to a weak contraction of the heart is called *systolic heart failure.* Diastole is the resting state of the heart when it is filled with blood. The inability of the heart to fill adequately with blood is then called *diastolic heart failure.*

Systolic heart failure results most often from arteriosclerotic heart disease. The patient has heart attacks which destroy the muscle of the heart or has chronic left ventricular volume overload due to valvular disease, especially mitral insufficiency, or a leaky mitral valve. A less common cause of systolic heart failure is failure of the heart muscle itself. This is called a cardiomyopathy. In either case, the muscle of the heart is weakened, the heart balloons in size and because of those changes it cannot contract efficiently.

Diastolic heart failure is akin to the weightlifter who lifts weights to make his muscles heftier. Unfortunately, hefty muscles may look good, but they do not contract very quickly. A wiry boxer is much more mobile than a hulk. Diastolic failure is due to too great an afterload. It occurs in the patient with long-standing hypertension or in the patient whose aortic valve is thickened and narrowed so blood cannot exit the left ventricle easily. The left ventricle has to work hard to expel the blood. If a patient has pulmonary hypertension the same changes occur in the right ventricle, and we say the patient has cor pulmonale. An unusual cause of diastolic heart muscle is due to thickening of the pericardial lining of the heart. The pericardium is a sac surrounding the heart. Thickening of the pericardium is most often due to a viral infection, tuberculosis, or cancer.

When the heart fails the cardiac output is decreased. This results in secondary changes which must also be addressed. The blood flow going to the kidneys is decreased resulting in a low glomerular filtration rate. The sensors in the kidneys interpret this as low blood volume and act to retain water by activating the renin-angiotensin-aldosterone system (RAAS). This results in the kidney reabsorbing more sodium and water and raising the preload or the diastolic filling of the heart. The low cardiac output is also sensed as low blood pressure by the carotid bodies. They activate the sympathetic nervous system causing the heart to beat faster and the blood pressure to rise increasing the afterload. Both effects give a short-term boost to the cardiac output but over time cause even more problems for the patient.

There is a third system that involves the heart muscle itself. The cardiac muscle, especially the muscle of the right atrium, contains a chemical called brain natriuretic peptide or ProBNP. There are two types: beta and alpha. Both B-type natriuretic peptide and A-type natriuretic peptide have beneficial hemodynamic effects during heart failure and represent a natural mechanism to relieve symptoms. They are released primarily in the atrium, as the elevated cardiac pressures stretch the atrial myocytes, are broken down to BNP, and act to cause vasodilation and cause sodium excretion by enhancing the glomerular filtration rate. In addition, the damaged heart releases Cardiac Troponin which has a similar effect as the BNP.

The activation of the RAAS causes fluid to accumulate everywhere in the body. The feet become swollen with salt and water, the liver engorged with fluid, and the lungs become edematous. The preload gets greater and greater and the cardiac muscle becomes overstretched. The stroke volume falls rather than increases with further increments to the preload. The activation of the sympathetic nervous raises the pulse rate and blood pressure. The tachycardia increases the need of the heart for more oxygen. But the tachycardia decreases the time in diastole and hence the filling of the coronary arteries. The increase in the blood pressure raises the afterload so the stroke volume falls even more. Thus, whatever benefit these changes made initially are soon vanquished.

The signs and symptoms we encounter in the patient with CHF are largely due to the activation of the RAAS and the sympathetic nervous system. The patient will be diaphoretic and tachycardic. He will be short of breath because of the fluid in his lungs. He may be cyanotic. He may have orthopnea, in which he is unable to lie down without becoming dyspneic. He may have paroxysmal nocturnal dyspnea or PND which is characterized by the patient awakening in the middle of the night extremely short of breath. He may have anorexia and muscle wasting due to liver engorgement. He may have pedal edema. The low cardiac output may also cause symptoms directly. The patient may be confused because his brain is not getting enough blood. His skin may be mottled because it is not getting enough blood.

Congestive heart failure is divided into four stages. Stage A is the "at risk" stage. This includes patients who are at risk of developing congestive heart failure. Patients with diabetes, hypercholesterolemia, hypertension, and obesity fall into this category. Stage B are those patients who have "pre-heart failure." These patients have cardiac enlargement, a problem with the heart muscle, or an abnormal heart valve. Often, they will have an increased BNP or Cardiac Troponin. The third group is the patient with "heart failure." These patients have symptoms or signs of heart failure. The last group, Stage D, are those patients with "advanced heart failure" who have severe symptoms and have had multiple hospitalizations of congestive heart failure. They need of a heart transplant or mechanical circulatory support.

The diagnosis of CHF rests upon finding the signs and symptoms consistent with the disease. More than 85% of patients with acute congestive heart failure have shortness of breath. It is the most common symptom of acute heart failure, but its specificity is only about 51%. Any patient with shortness of breath and any of the other signs or symptoms of congestive heart failure should have a chest radiograph. The chest x-ray is often diagnostic. Findings include cephalization of blood flow (the arteries at the top of the lung are distended), diffuse interstitial changes, Kerley B lines (thin, short horizontal lines arising from the pleural surface at the lung bases), and pleural effusions. The heart will be enlarged if the patient has systolic heart failure and normal in size if the patient has diastolic dysfunction. In severe and very acute cases the interstitial changes may have a "butterfly" or "batwing" appearance.

Patients with chronic heart failure may state that they are short of breath because they are chair bound and don't do anything to make them dyspneic. They present with fatigue, anorexia (loss of appetite), abdominal distention, and pedal edema.

If the chest x-ray is suggestive of congestive heart failure, a BNP or brain naturetic peptide should be done along with a complete blood count and chemistry panel which includes electrolytes, renal function, liver function, and glucose. An EKG is necessary as well. The BNP will be more than 300 pgrams/l in a patient in the emergency room with congestive heart failure. However, severe COPD or a pulmonary embolism can cause false positives by causing right heart failure. False negatives can occur as well. The normal outpatient value for BNP is less than 35 pgrams/l.

The complete blood count may be helpful. Severe anemia (low hemoglobin) can precipitate congestive heart failure. The chemistry panel is needed to evaluate renal or kidney function. Are the kidneys impaired? In addition, because patients with congestive heart failure are retaining water and salt because of the hormone aldosterone, the potassium may be low making patient more at risk of serious cardiac arrhythmias.

The electrocardiogram will demonstrate the presence of any arrhythmias and can also show signs of a prior myocardial infarction or changes due to severe hypertension.

Once the diagnosis of CHF is established, the most important test to perform is the echocardiogram. The echocardiogram is done to determine the type of CHF HFrEF versus HFpEF) and the severity of the condition. The echocardiogram is a micro-radar device. It can measure the thickness of the walls of the heart. It can also measure how the cardiac valves function. In addition, it can measure blood flow and from the measured blood flow calculate the cardiac output. Thus, it can readily differentiate between systolic and diastolic heart failure which is critical to the care of the patient. The patient with systolic dysfunction (HFrEF) will have a dilated left ventricle with poor contraction. There may even be parts of the ventricle which do not contract at all. If the CHF is severe, there may be severe back flow of blood through a dilated mitral valve. In any case, the left ventricular ejection fraction (the amount of blood ejected on each beat divided by the left ventricular end diastolic volume) will be markedly reduced. On the other hand, the patient with diastolic CHF (HFpEF) will have a thickened left ventricular wall and a hyper-dynamic heart. The ejection fraction will, in fact, be normal.

Lastly, in the critically ill patient in which the diagnosis is still unsure or if help is needed to guide therapy, a right-heart catheterization using a Swan-Ganz catheter can be used. This is a long multi-channeled catheter that is inserted into the heart and pulmonary arteries vis the internal jugular vein or the right subclavian vein. The catheter has a balloon near its tip which can be inflated to help guide the catheter during insertion. It also has a channel for measuring pressure. It is threaded with the balloon inflated into the superior vena cava, thence to the right atrium, right ventricle, and pulmonary artery. Finally, the catheter tip is placed in a segmental pulmonary artery. When the balloon is inflated it will stop the blood flow in the segmental artery. Thus, there will be no flow distal to the balloon. The pressure at the tip of the balloon will be the same as in the pulmonary vein. During diastole, there is no blood flow in the heart. The heart is at rest and the mitral valve is open. Thus, *since there is no blood flow between the catheter and the left ventricle, the pressure in the left ventricle is the same as the pressure in the left atrium, is the same as the pressure in the pulmonary veins, and is the same as the pressure at the tip of the catheter.* This pressure is called the **Left Ventricular End Diastolic Pressure** (LVEDP) and is a measure of the preload. The normal value is less than 18 mm Hg. If the pressure is greater than this, the preload is too great, and the patient is in heart failure. The LVEDP can be used to guide therapy including the use of diuretics. Thus, both too little and too much diuresis can be avoided.

Complications resulting from the placement of the Swan-Ganz catheter include perforation of the right ventricle resulting in blood spilling into the pericardium and squeezing the heart, a condition called cardiac tamponade. The catheter may also cause serious and even fatal cardiac arrhythmias. In addition, if the balloon is left inflated for too long a time, a blood clot may form distal to the catheter.

The treatment of congestive heart failure, both systolic and diastolic, begins with life-style changes. The patient needs to quit smoking. He or she needs to refrain from alcohol. Even one Martini decreases the strength of a cardiac contraction. The patient should be instructed in a Mediterranean diet and be given an exercise program. Every patient with pre heart disease or heart disease should be treated with medication to lower the cholesterol such as Lipitor or Crestor. Sodium intake should be restricted to less than three grams a day and fluid should be restricted to less than two liters a day. Diabetes and hypertension must be treated aggressively. Weight should be monitored to ensure that the patient is not retaining fluid.

Any underlying condition should be treated. Does the patient have ischemic heart disease due to atherosclerosis? A left-heart cardiac catheterization examining the coronary arteries may need to be done to see if there is any blockage. Does the patient have a diseased heart valve? The echocardiogram should be able to detect a diseased mitral or aortic valve which may need to be repaired or replaced. Does the patient have a cardiac arrhythmia such as atrial fibrillation? Medication may be needed to control the heart rate. Is the patient anemic? If so, the cause of the anemia should be determined, and the anemia corrected. Low hemoglobin will put a lot of stress on a failing heart. In fact, some patients with pernicious anemia due to B12 deficiency can have a hemoglobin of less than 6 and go into heart failure just due to the anemia alone. Does the patient have sleep apnea? Does the patient have hypoxemia?

If the patient is African American, test should be done for the aTTR gene which causes amyloidosis of the heart. The gene is present in 4-5% of blacks. Recently, medical therapy to treat the disorder has been developed but the disease must be caught early when the patient is in his 40's and not when he is in his 60's with severe heart disease.

The treatment of the patient with systolic dysfunction, which accounts for half the patients with congestive heart failure, addresses the three cardiac parameters we already mentioned: the preload, the afterload, and the contractility. The most important first step in treating the patient with mild to moderate congestive heart failure is to address the afterload. If the afterload is decreased, the work the heart must do is decreased and the cardiac output (or stroke volume) will increase. Medicines that decrease the blood pressure, specifically the angiotensin converting enzyme inhibitors (ACE inhibitors) such as Vasotec or Captopril and the angiotensin receptor blockers (ARB) such as Diovan, are the best choices. Both classes of medications block the RAAS system. In the patient with severe congestive heart failure and high blood pressure intravenous nitroglycerin or nitroprusside can be used instead. Both agents also reduce the preload.

If reducing the afterload is not enough decreasing the preload is the next step. This is generally done with diuretics such as furosemide or with medicines that dilate the great veins such as intravenous nitroprusside or nitroglycerin. Another choice not often used as much anymore unfortunately is intravenous morphine sulfate. This agent lowers the blood pressure, the preload, and relieves anxiety thus decreasing the sympathetic nervous system effects. Using the medication for one day will not addict the patient.

Finally, in critically ill patients, medications that increase the contractility can be tried. These are all essentially adrenergic agents such as dopamine. The downside to increasing the contractility is that this increases the oxygen demands of the heart dramatically. Both reducing the afterload and preload do not.

Other medications that are used to treat systolic congestive heart failure include the aldosterone antagonists (spironolactone) also known as "potassium sparing diuretics" or MRAs (mineralocorticoid receptor antagonists), which block the action of aldosterone, inhibiting the reuptake of sodium and water by the kidney. As sodium is reabsorbed, it is exchanged with a potassium molecule, which is then excreted resulting in hypokalemia. Aldosterone inhibition decreases sodium and water reabsorption and decreases potassium excretion, resulting in improvement in fluid balance but with the risk of hyperkalemia.

The current Guideline Directed Medical Therapy or GDMT includes an ARNI (an ARB and a neprilysin inhibitor taken together. The neprilysin inhibitors increase guanyl cyclase levels and help prevent scarring or fibrosis of the heart), a B blocker, an MRA such as spironolactone, and a diuretic such as furosemide if needed. The most recent guidelines suggest that a SLGT2 inhibitor should be added. This class of medicine blocks the reabsorption of sugar in the kidney. Thus, sugar is excreted in the urine taking water with it. This improves the preload of the heart. In addition, the medication lowers the sugar and improves cardiac metabolism. A new agent, Vericiguat, increases the sensitivity to nitrous oxide (NO), stimulating guanyl cyclase and increasing GMP (guanyl-monophosphate). This action causes smooth muscle relaxation, vasodilation, and improved cardiac function.

Other therapies include oxygen, non-invasive ventilation if needed and even intubation. The use of ECMO (extracorporeal membrane oxygenation) as a temporary bridge to a heart transplant is being used more often.

Some patients with end-stage congestive heart failure may benefit from an implantable cardiac defibrillator. Most patients with CHF die of ventricular arrhythmias and if ventricular tachycardia can be caught early and treated the patient will live longer.

Lastly, surgery may be helpful in certain patients with systolic heart failure. These surgeries include removing a left ventricular aneurysm (a dead piece of the wall of the left ventricle) or doing a cardiac transplant if the patient is young and healthy enough, implanting a cardiac assist device, or lastly doing a mitral valve repair via a femoral vein catheter. The latter surgery involves partially stapling the leaflets of the mitral valve together to reduce the degree of mitral insufficiency which is both major complication of a dilated left ventricle and a condition which makes congestive heart failure even worse.

In the past diastolic heart failure was considered much more difficult to treat, Treatment, in general, was unsatisfactory. No treatment prolonged life expectancy. Once CHF set in in a patient with hypertensive heart disease, the course of the disease was set. Recent evidence suggests that the life expectancy of patients with preserved ejection fraction is the same as those with reduced ejection fraction and the treatment of the two conditions is the same

The treatment of hypertension in Blacks is more complex. Blacks tend to have a low renin level. Thus, they have excess effective circulating blood volume as the cause of their hypertension. Because of this, diuretics, and certain Calcium Channel Blockers (including Amlodipine and Nifedipine) are the first lines of therapy.

If the patient has aortic stenosis (narrowing of the opening of the aortic valve) as a cause of his or her diastolic heart failure, then the treatment is to replace the aortic valve. The newest approach is via a catheter placed in the femoral artery and threaded back to the heart. The new valve is inserted over the old diseased valve. The surgery is indicated in patients with moderate and severe aortic stenosis. The main side effect is the development of atrial fibrillation after the valve is placed. But the results of the catheter placed aortic valve replacement (TAVR) are as good as those of the surgically replaced aortic valves.

The last case presentation was a patient with thickening of the pericardium due to tuberculosis. This is certainly a very uncommon cause of "diastolic cardiac dysfunction." The pericardial sac is to the heart as the pleural sac is to the lungs. It has both a visceral and parietal surface, the latter is the outer layer of the heart, covering the heart muscle. The sac has only a scanty amount of fluid normally.

However, several conditions can cause the sac to become inflamed and filled with fluid or blood. Certainly, the most common is acute viral pericarditis, which is often seen in a young, otherwise healthy individual and while quite painful is generally short-lived without long-term consequences.

But there are many causes of acute and chronic pericarditis including bacterial infections, tuberculosis, and aspergillosis in patients with AIDS, the collagen vascular diseases including systemic lupus erythematosus and rheumatoid arthritis, chronic renal disease, and chest wall trauma especially trauma due to a steering wheel and radiation.

Most often the symptoms of acute pericarditis include fever and chest pain. The pain is sharp and localized either substernally or to the left of the sternum. It radiates towards the left shoulder and feels better sitting up and leaning forward but worse lying down. If there is a large amount of fluid or blood in the sac which impairs the diastolic function of the heart, symptoms and signs of cardiac failure will also be seen. Auscultation of the heart during the physical exam of the patient with acute pericarditis often shows a "crunching" sound like the "creaking of leather boots" or a "scratchy" sound like leaves in a breeze with each heartbeat. The combination of the type of chest pain and the auscultatory findings are classic.

The electrocardiogram is often diagnostic showing diffuse elevation of the ST segment. The echocardiogram is also helpful demonstrating thickening of the pericardium or fluid in the pericardial space. Treatment depends totally on the underlying cause.

An acute life-threatening cause of acute pericarditis is due to the perforation of the right ventricular wall occurring during the placement of the Swan-Ganz. This is a surgical emergency.

Chronic pericarditis is most often due to cancer invading the pericardium or to tuberculosis. A pericardiocentesis (removing fluid from the pericardial sac) needs to be done to determine the cause. The symptoms are generally those of diastolic heart failure although the patient with cancer may have serious cardiac arrhythmias as well. Again, the treatment depends upon the cause.

Suggestions for Minor Papers

1. What is the relationship between congestive heart failure and sleep apnea?
2. Why do patients with atrial fibrillation need anticoagulants?
3. Compare systolic and diastolic heart failure.
4. Compare backward and forward congestive heart failure
5. Explain the RAAS system.
6. Where does BNP come from?
7. What are the causes of atherosclerosis?

Seven

Diffuse Parenchymal Lung Disease

The interstitial lung diseases include more than a hundred and fifty different disorders of various pathologies bound together because they are diseases of the lung parenchyma and are restrictive lung diseases. Some also involve the pulmonary vasculature such as Wegener's Granulomatosis (Granulomatosis with Polyangiitis). Some are peribronchial diseases such as Sarcoidosis. Some are diseases of alveoli and surrounding interstitial tissue such as Usual Interstitial Pneumonitis. They differ so much from one another that it is exceedingly difficult to place them all in one basket. They are, in essence, a potpourri of diseases.

The four most commonly encountered interstitial diseases are Usual Interstitial Pneumonitis or UIP, Non-specific Interstitial Pneumonitis or NSIP, Sarcoidosis, and Hypersensitivity Pneumonitis (HP). Each of these illnesses has a different clinical presentation, a different pathology, a different therapy, and a different eventual outcome. Two occupational diseases must be discussed as well, even though they are seen much less frequently today. These are Asbestosis and Silicosis.

Usual Interstitial Pneumonitis is a disease of old age. The typical patient is in a man in his sixties or older. Often the patient is an ex-smoker. The hallmark of the disease is subpleural fibrosis with honeycombing. Fibrosis is the main feature, and it is dramatic. The disease progresses rapidly, the patient dying within four years. *Nonspecific Interstitial Pneumonitis,* on the other hand, occurs in patients in their fifties. While the disease is also subpleural there isn't any honeycombing, and the lungs have a "ground glass" appearance suggesting active inflammation. The disease is progressive but does respond to corticosteroids and the patient can live well over a decade. *Sarcoidosis* is a disease of unknown origin characterized by the presence of peribronchial "granulomata" throughout the lung. The cause of the disease is unknown. Most patients don't require any treatment at all. *Hypersensitivy Pneumonitis* is an inflammatory interstitial process caused by an antibody response to various antigens ranging from bird dander to heat-loving bacteria. While the occupational disorders are much less common today in the United States, they may still be encountered in patients from overseas, especially Africa and Asia, where asbestos and silica are still used, often without much regulation.

Peter A. Petroff, MD

Case Presentations

1.

Enrique T. is a 72-year-old male who comes to the outpatient pulmonary clinic complaining of cough and shortness of breath. He states he has been ill for about a year or a little more. The illness began with shortness of breath which has gradually gotten worse. He tells the doctor that a year ago he played soccer with his grandchildren but a few months ago he had to give it up. Since then, the shortness of breath has gotten much worse. He also noted that he began having a dry, irritating cough about six months ago. He states, "The cough is far worse than the breathing doc." The cough is unremitting, night and day. Three months ago, he went to his family doctor who told him to quit smoking. He did but the cough has not changed. In fact, it is worse.

The patient states he smoked about a pack a day for fifty years. He drinks a couple of beers once a week. He takes an over-the-counter cough medicine which has not helped. He is not allergic to any medicines. He has not had any surgery or medical admissions. He worked as an auto mechanic and gardener all his adult life. He has not travelled outside the city in more than ten years.

His physical examination shows him to be an alert thin male who is short of breath with any exertion. His BP is 146/72; Pulse is 76; Height is 5'10"; Weight is 176 lbs.; he is afebrile. His examination is normal except for mild cyanosis, early clubbing, poor chest expansion, slight generalized dullness to percussion, decreased breath sounds with fine inspiratory crackles over the lower lobes, slight liver enlargement, and trace pedal edema.

The chest x-ray shows bibasilar interstitial infiltrates with prominent hila without cardiac enlargement.

The laboratory findings, including a CBC and chemistry profile, are normal. Testing for autoimmune disease is negative as well. His PPD is negative.

The patient is sent for a High-Resolution CAT scan of the chest (HRCT) which showed bilateral basilar subpleural fibrotic changes associated with honeycombing as well as traction diverticular changes of the small airways. The radiologist stated that the findings were diagnostic for UIP or Usual Interstitial Pneumonitis.

After the study Enrique and his wife met with the pulmonologist who suggested that, while they could do a biopsy to be absolutely sure, it wasn't really necessary. The HRCT was enough to make a diagnosis in view of the fact that Enrique never worked with asbestos and the studies for autoimmune disease were normal. Instead, the physician recommended getting pulmonary function testing, which would serve as a baseline, and then beginning therapy. He also recommended a transesophageal echocardiogram to look for signs of pulmonary hypertension and a six-minute walk.

The PFTs were as follows:

FVC	72% of predicted
FEV1	74% of predicted
MMF	75% of predicted
TLC	72% of predicted
RV	78% of predicted
DCO	42% of predicted

There was no evidence of pulmonary hypertension. The six-minute walk showed significant loss of function. The normal distance a 55-75-year-old could walk in six minutes is between 500 and 800 meters. Enrique could only walk 30 meters. Even then his SaO2 dropped from 88% to 82% with the exercise.

The doctor offered Enrique two choices of medications: Nintedanib and Pirfenidone. The only other therapy was a lung transplant and the doctor said he would refer Enrique to the lung transplant group at the clinic now rather than waiting to see how he does with the medication. He also began him on oxygen at 2 l/minutes per nasal cannula and scheduled a sleep study.

Nintedanib was begun at 150 mg twice a day taken with food. Almost immediately, Enrique developed diarrhea. The doctor said that this was the main side effect of the drug and told him to stop the medication if the diarrhea was too much a problem. Enrique stopped the medication.

Enrique then began taking Pirfenidone at 800 mg a day, increasing it to 2400 mg a day over the next three weeks. At first, he had some nausea but gradually he felt better and was able to tolerate the medication. While the shortness of breath did not improve, it also did not worsen. The cough remained unchanged. After six months the PFTs were repeated:

FVC	70% of predicted
FEV1	74% of predicted
MMF	75% of predicted
TLC	74% of predicted
RV	78% of predicted
DCO	34% of predicted

The lung volumes were stable though the diffusing capacity worsened slightly. The medication was continued while Enrique awaited a lung transplant.

2.

Sarah C. is a 24-year-old Black woman who visits the pulmonary clinic with an unremitting cough. She tells the doctor she has had the cough for six months. She saw her primary doctor who did a chest x-ray which was "normal." He began her on an antibiotic, but it did not help. She was referred to an allergist because her doctor heard some wheezing. The allergist did "breathing tests" which were "pretty normal" and did an allergy "prick test" panel which was also normal. He then started her on an albuterol inhaler, but it has not helped at all. She decided to see a lung specialist on her own.

The cough is an irritating cough. It is generally dry but occasionally she has some clear phlegm. She has noted a few wheezes at times, but the wheezing is not constant. She is not short of breath unless she hurries up a flight of stairs. She has no fever, chills, or night sweats.

Sarah's past history is unremarkable. She has never smoked or "vaped." She does not take any recreational drugs such as alcohol, cocaine, or marijuana. She has no drug allergies. She has not had any surgery or medical admissions. She is single and lives in an apartment in the city. She works as a personal secretary to the president of a large industrial company. She enjoys her work. Her only hobby is reading.

Her physical examination shows her to be alert and in no distress. Her BP is 110/60; pulse is 74; height is 5'4"; weight is 124 lbs. The doctor noted a couple of darkish brown papules on her legs. The patient was not aware of them.

The examination of her head and neck is unremarkable. The lungs were clear with normal breath sounds. The heart showed an occasional ectopic beat, probably a paroxysmal ventricular contraction. The liver was normal in size. The spleen was not palpable. There was no edema.

The doctor ordered a chest radiograph, CBC, chemistry profile, sedimentation rate, and C-reactive protein as well as pulmonary function testing.

The chest x-ray showed bilateral hilar enlargement. The right hilum, while enlarged, did not encroach on the right heart border. The laboratory was all normal. The pulmonary function testing was as follows:

FVC 86% of predicted
FEV1 72% of predicted
MMF 65% of predicted
TLC 88% of predicted
RV 90% of predicted
DCO 64% of predicted

The studies were consistent with a mild obstructive disease associated with decreased diffusion.

Sarah returned to the clinic after the studies were completed. The doctor told Sarah he believed she had Sarcoidosis. He explained to her that it was a disease of unknown cause and that for most patients the disease need not be treated because it would resolve over a few years on its own. He based his diagnosis on the chest radiograph showing the symmetrical hilar enlargement.

He was concerned, however, because of her cough and suggested that she get a HRCT scan which was done. The HRCT confirmed the findings of the chest x-ray and did not show any signs of parenchymal involvement. But, because of her cough, he advised her to get a transbronchoscopic lung biopsy. Sarah agreed.

The transbronchoscopic lung biopsy showed small non-caseous granulomas in the lung parenchyma. Sarah was begun on high dose corticosteroids (1 mg/kg/day). The cough disappeared within a few weeks. After three months the dose was tapered and finally stopped after 9 months. The cough did not recur. The chest radiograph, however, remained unchanged, again showing the bilateral hilar enlargement. A dermatologist biopsied one of the skin lesions. The biopsy was also consistent with sarcoidosis. The dose of corticosteroids was decreased after one month and then tapered slowly over nine months.

3.

Alfonse T. is an 83-year-old male who visits the pulmonary clinic because of severe shortness of breath. The patient states that he has been short of breath for years, "At least ten years, maybe more." The shortness of breath is getting worse. He cannot walk more than 10 feet without dyspnea. He has a little cough with clear phlegm. He has never coughed up blood. He has not had any chest pain or pressure in his chest. Nor has he had any orthopnea or pedal edema. He is fine when he sits watching TV.

He has never smoked. He does not drink or use recreational drugs. He does not take any medication and has no drug allergies. He has never been near a hospital except when his wife or his kids had kids. His review of systems is surprisingly unremarkable. Both his parents died of what the doctors called "congestive heart failure."

His social history is important. He was born in Monterrey, Mexico and came to Austin when he was 6 years of age. His father was a painter and began working for a major homebuilder within days of their move to Austin. Alfonse did well in school but when he graduated from high school in 1952, he became a painter, just like his father. He did residential and light industrial construction. After six years he became a foreman and then in 1986 became vice president of the construction company. He continued to work there until he retired in 2007 at the age of 73.

As a painter he painted walls and cabinets. He also "taped and floated" wall board. He used Gold-Bond sealant almost daily from 1952 to 1976 when it was discontinued.

The shortness of breath began about 1996. At first it was mild but then it got worse and worse. "It was just like my father and mother," Alfonse told the doctor. The doctor asked Alfonse if his mother washed his father's clothing. Alfonse answered, "Yes, almost every day. The clothes were always coated in this gray stuff. It was more than just paint."

The physical exam showed Alfonse to be mildly obese but in no distress while sitting comfortably. His BP was 104/78; his pulse was 102; his height was 5'8"; his weight was 186 lbs. His SaO2 at rest was 88%. There was no obvious cyanosis. There was no clubbing.

His lungs showed bibasilar inspiratory crackles. The rest of the exam was totally normal.

The doctor ordered a chest radiograph which showed a bibasilar reticular interstitial disease consistent with pulmonary fibrosis. The left heart border was indistinct. The radiologist called it the "shaggy heart sign." There were many small, calcified plaques along the pleural surface as well. The heart was normal in size. There were no signs of congestive heart failure.

The doctor told Alfonse that he had asbestosis with asbestos pleural disease. Because he was 83, he did not think he could tolerate a lung transplant, but he would send him to see the transplant team anyway to get their opinion. He also began him on oxygen at 2 l/minute per nasal cannula.

The doctor ordered routine testing including a CBC, chemistry profile, urinalysis, BPH and C-reactive protein, all of which were normal as expected.

Alfonse asked the doctor if he should have a biopsy to prove it was asbestosis. The doctor said he saw absolutely no reason for the biopsy. The diagnosis was certain.

Background for the presentations

UIP is a disease of aging. The older you are the more likely you are to get it. It might be called the "Alzheimer's disease of the lung." In about 10% of cases, it is due to a heritable genetic abnormality. The disease is progressive with death occurring in just 4-5 years. The newest medications slow the deterioration of pulmonary function but don't cure it.

Sarcoidosis is usually a restrictive disease but occasionally can present as an obstructive disease if the bronchi are diseased. Cough and wheezing can be a symptom though usually the patient is asymptomatic. The key to making a diagnosis of asbestosis is taking a good history, doing a good examination, and getting a chest radiograph and, often, a high resolution CAT scan of the chest.

Asbestos is a due to exposure to the asbestos fiber. It is most often seen in painters, insulators, boilermakers, and electricians who worked in the era before the mid 1970's. It causes symptoms and signs similar to UIP, but clubbing is much less likely and should prompt a search for cancer which is also a well-known complication of asbestos exposure.

Important points

1. UIP can be diagnosed just on the HRCT if the findings are typical.
2. Treatment in the past for UIP included steroids and anti-inflammatory agents which actually hastened the demise of the patient.
3. The course of UIP is a *stepwise* descent to respiratory failure, rather than a continuous decline.
4. Sarcoidosis is multi-systemic involving the lungs, skin, eyes, heart, and liver.

5. Sarcoidosis can present with either a restrictive disease pattern or an obstructive disease pattern. However, diffusion is almost always impaired.
6. Sarcoidosis is most commonly seen in Blacks in the United States, but outside of the US, Caucasians are just as susceptible.
7. Ten percent of patients with Sarcoidosis go on to develop classic emphysema.
8. The only way to make a diagnosis of a pneumoconiosis is to take a thorough work history.

Discussion

There are over a hundred and fifty types of Idiopathic Pulmonary Fibrosis (IPF). What do they have in common? But can all the disorders be characterized as some "type" of pulmonary fibrosis? Are they all restrictive diseases?

No, not all the disorders have pulmonary fibrosis as their primary pathologic finding. Some do, including Usual Interstitial Pneumonitis-Fibrosis (UIP), non-specific interstitial pulmonary disease (NSIP) and Asbestosis. But Sarcoidosis and Pulmonary Alveolar Proteinosis (PAP) do not, at least in their early stages. It is true that most of the diseases included in the category IPF have a restrictive disease pattern on their pulmonary function. But Sarcoidosis and Asbestosis, at least early on, may have an obstructive pattern. One unifying pattern might be the diffusing capacity, which is reduced to a greater or lesser extent in almost all of the diseases in this group.

Because of this, the name of this group of diseases has recently been changed from Idiopathic Pulmonary Fibrosis to **Diffuse Parenchymal Lung Disease** (DPLD) which makes much more sense.

Classifying the diseases is even more difficult. Some, like Asbestosis, have a known cause. Most, like Sarcoidosis, don't. Some, like UIP, NSIP, pulmonary fibrosis due to certain drugs such as Cytoxan and Methotrexate, as well as Asbestosis, involve primarily the lower lung fields while some, like Sarcoidosis, Hypersensitivity Pneumonitis, and Silicosis, involve the upper lobes primarily. Some are characterized as fibrotic, some are characterized as granulomatous, and still others as a vasculitis, and some even as a vasculitis with granulomatous features. Some like UIP can have associated pulmonary hypertension though most don't. Because of that, it is easier to concentrate on the common disorders which may or may not need a lung biopsy to make the diagnosis and lump the less common ones into groups that generally require a lung biopsy.

One classification that I like:

> Known etiology
> > Occupational Diseases or pneumoconiosis
> > Inhaled organic dusts (Hypersensitivity Pneumonitis)
> > Iatrogenic (due to certain medications or radiation)
> Unknown etiology
> > Usual interstitial pneumonitis
> > Non-Specific interstitial pneumonitis including autoimmune disorders
> > Sarcoidosis

Less common
    Goodpasture's disease
    Granulomatosis with Polyangiitis (Wegener's Granulomatosis)
    Pulmonary Alveolar Proteinosis
    Chronic eosinophilic pneumonitis

Almost all of the diseases have two things in common. The first and foremost is inflammation involving the alveolar wall and the alveolar spaces. The second is some form of scarring or fibrosis. Some of the pathologies such as Sarcoidosis are characterized by granulomata. A granuloma is a nodular collection of phagocytic epithelial histiocytes associated with T lymphocytes and giant cells which are large, multinuclear cells derived from the macrophages.

The four most common causes of Diffuse Parenchymal Lung Disease (DPLD) are Usual Interstitial Pneumonitis-Fibrosis (UIP), Non-Specific Interstitial Pneumonitis-Fibrosis (NSIP), Sarcoidosis, and Hypersensitivity Pneumonitis (HP). Each has a different etiology, epidemiology, clinical presentation, pathology, and treatment. As a whole these four disorders account for about 80% of cases of Diffuse Parenchymal Lung Disease. Each of them can usually be diagnosed without the need for a lung biopsy. The most common occupational diseases are Asbestosis and Silicosis. Both of these are diagnosed solely on the history and clinical findings including radiology.

The pathophysiology of most of these diseases includes stiff lungs with decreased compliance, small airway dysfunction, decreased alveolar-capillary surface area, and, in some cases, pulmonary hypertension. Hypoxemia without hypercapnia is the rule and is most often due to ventilation-perfusion inequality. In the patient with end stage disease some CO_2 retention may occur as well. Most patients have a restrictive defect on their pulmonary function with decreased TLC, slightly decreased RV and decreased FRC but some patients have an obstructive pattern due to small airways disease and some have a mixed restrictive and obstructive pattern. Diffusion is usually decreased as well because of the destruction of the capillary bed and increased heart rate due to hypoxemia which decreases the time blood spends in the pulmonary capillaries. Exercise, by further shortening the time the blood is in the capillary, will magnify the diffusion abnormality.

The most common symptom of all the diffuse parenchymal disease is shortness of breath. The presence of shortness of breath suggests the need for a chest radiograph which will likely show the interstitial prominence and may show signs of pulmonary hypertension as well. The patient is then sent for a high-resolution CAT scan of the chest which is often diagnostic. If it is not, then a lung biopsy needs to be done. If Sarcoidosis is suspected the biopsy can be done through a bronchoscope; if not, then an open lung biopsy needs to be done.

Usual Interstitial Pneumonitis Fibrosis is a disease of unknown etiology although recent studies suggest that it is likely caused by an abnormality of the genetic makeup which causes dysfunctional lung repair after an injury. 10% of patients have hereditary UIP while 90% of patients have spontaneous or idiopathic UIP. Recent evidence has shown that between 19% and 31% of relatives of patients with UIP, whether sporadic or familial, have early evidence of interstitial lung abnormalities. The risk of UIP in these relatives is worse with increased age, decreased FVC or DCO, decreased length of telomeres in lymphocytes, male sex, and smoking. This finding is important because the use of antifibrotics is more effective in patients with early disease and preserved lung function. It is important to diagnose UIP as early as possible. One researcher suggested strongly that all first-degree relatives of patients with UIP should be screened for the disease with PFTs and chest radiographs.

The disease is more commonly seen in smokers or ex-smokers. It is a disease of men predominantly. The typical patient used to be a man in his late 60's or early 70's. But now, it is clear, that the older you are the more likely you are to get UIP. Like Alzheimer's disease, it is a disease of aging. Many believe that the disease occurs because of abnormal healing resulting in fibrosis which follows an inflammation of the alveoli resulting in disruption of the alveolar basement membrane.

The disease presents with shortness of breath and a dry, irritating, unremitting cough. For some patients, the cough is much more a problem than the breathing. Clinical findings include hypoxemia with a decreased SaO2 especially with exercise, bilateral basilar inspiratory crackles, also known as "Velcro Rales," and sometimes clubbing of the fingers. The chest radiograph shows bilateral basilar reticular changes consistent with fibrosis and the pulmonary function testing shows a restrictive disease pattern with a marked decrease in the diffusion capacity.

The disease can be diagnosed on the HRCT alone. If there are bilateral lower lobe sub-pleural reticular interstitial changes associated with the presence of "honeycombing" or large and small cystic lesions, as well as traction diverticula extending from the small bronchi, but most importantly, there is be no signs of a "ground glass appearance," a sign of active inflammation, the diagnosis is established. No biopsy need be done. Treatment can begin at once. The only problem would be if the patient worked with asbestos which could be confused with UIP on x-ray. However, asbestosis is usually, but not necessarily, accompanied by pleural changes. In addition, of course, there is a history of exposure to the asbestos fiber.

The prognosis of UIP is grim. The life expectancy after diagnosis is no more than four years. The course of the disease is marked by acute exacerbations with a step-like decline in function rather than a steady unremitting downhill progression. The patient will be stable for months then suddenly have an exacerbation which irreversibly worsens his condition. The causes of the exacerbations are unknown. They may be episodes of viral pneumonia. Typically, the high-resolution CAT scan will show a ground glass appearance consistent with an alveolitis during an exacerbation.

The treatment in the past relied on steroids and anti-cancer agents like Cytoxan. But, as it turns out, steroids and medications like Cytoxan actually make the condition worse. In the last two years two new agents have been described: Nintedanib and pirfenidone. Both are anti-fibrinogenic. They slow the decline in pulmonary function testing but do not reverse the disease process itself. Recently, a new therapy, phosphodiesterase 4b, which prevents the proliferation and differentiation of fibroblasts has shown impressive results. In a phase 2 study published in 2022, (a study done to test the safety of the treatment), there was no change in the FVC at 12 weeks in patients treated with the agent, whereas the controls showed a decrease of 82 ccs.[3]

At present the only highly recommended treatments for IPF are oxygen and a lung transplant. Treatments with a moderate recommendation include Nintedanib and Pirfenidone as well as medications for gastric reflux such as Protonix.

All patients, if they are relatively healthy, should be sent to the transplant team for consideration of a lung transplant as soon as possible. In addition, all patients must be evaluated for the presence of pulmonary hypertension which often accompanies the disease.

In the chapter about pneumonia, we spoke about the lung biome. Of interest, recent studies have shown that even before there is an inflammatory reaction that will result in pulmonary fibrosis, there is a change in the biome. In fact, the type of bacteria present in the biome can predict the rate of progression of IPF!

Non-specific interstitial pneumonitis-fibrosis (NSIP) occurs in younger individuals. Like UIP it involves the lower lung fields predominantly. It differs from UIP in the findings on high resolution CAT scan, the course of the disease, and the response to steroids. The disease generally occurs in men and women in their fifties. The HRCAT scan shows only a small amount of fibrotic scarring. Instead, there is a ground glass appearance consistent with active alveolitis. The condition is associated with autoimmune diseases such as rheumatoid arthritis, scleroderma, and systemic lupus erythematosus. The disease often responds to steroids. The patient with NSIP may live for a decade or more with treatment. I know one patient that has lived, and doing well, for more than 20 years.

Sarcoidosis is a systemic disease of unknown etiology, often involving the skin, eyes, heart, and liver as well as the lungs. It is characterized by the presence of "non-caseating granulomas" which means the granulomas are solid, not cheesy like the granulomas found in tuberculosis and fungal infections. They do not have a necrotic center. Many different diseases such as tuberculosis, Berylliosis, and certain fungal diseases also cause granulomas. Interestingly, first responders to the attack at the World Trade Center attack in New York City also developed a granulomatous disease. Lastly, barium, zirconium, and the rare earth metals can cause granulomas. All these diseases must be excluded in order to establish a diagnosis of Sarcoidosis with absolute certainty. A thorough history is the key!

The disease generally occurs in younger patients, especially women and generally is self-limited. It occurs predominantly in Blacks in the US, but it involves mainly Puerto Ricans in New York City and in Whites in the Nordic countries. It can also occur in older people and, in that case, is often a fatal disease. The prevalence of Sarcoidosis is highest in Sweden, followed by Switzerland, Blacks in the United States, and Finland. The countries in northern Europe are most affected by the disease in

---

[3] Luca Richeldi, MD, PHD; NEJM 2022; 386: 2178-87

fact! Health care workers have an increased risk. The disease can even be transmitted by cardiac or bone marrow transplantation. Despite this, the cause of the disorder remains unknown.

The granulomas have an abundance of "CD4 helper cells with a Th1 profile." This results in activation of the inflammatory pathway in the tissue which results in the granulomas.

Typically, the patient presents because a routine chest radiograph was found to be abnormal, most often showing bilateral hilar adenopathy. The patient may also present with shortness of breath or a cough. Some patients present with painful red nodules on their extremities (erythema nodosum) associated with fever and bilateral hilar enlargement. This condition is called Löfgren Syndrome. Some patients present with cardiac abnormalities such as a cardiac arrhythmia. Some patients present with changes in their vision or iritis, an inflammation of the iris.

There are four stages of Sarcoidosis as shown chest radiographs.

1. The first is bilateral hilar adenopathy. This can be confused with a lymphoma or cancer of the lymphatic tissue, but in patients with Sarcoidosis there is a clear space between the right heart border and the right hilum.
2. The second stage is the presence of a diffuse interstitial process involving predominantly the upper lung fields.
3. The third is a combination of stage one and two.
4. The last stage is a patient whose chest radiograph looks like severe emphysematous disease.

If the patient has only hilar adenopathy, normal pulmonary function testing, and no findings to suggest eye or heart disease, no further work-up is needed. The patient can simply be followed. If on the other hand, the patient has parenchymal lung disease or restrictive lung disease or has cardiac or eye disease, a lung biopsy via the fiberoptic bronchoscope should be done. If the diagnosis is confirmed, then corticosteroids should be started. If the patient fails steroids, then an anti-inflammatory agent such as infliximab, an antagonist of tumor necrosis factor, can be tried. Methotrexate, an agent used in rheumatoid arthritis, can also be tried.

Hypersensitivity Pneumonitis is also known as extrinsic allergic alveolitis. It is an immunologic reaction to an inhaled antigen, most often an organic antigen, though inorganic antigens can bind to proteins and cause the reaction as well.

The earliest cases of HP were in farmers. The farmers in the northern part of our country cut hay during the summer and store it in their barns. Come winter, the cattle need to be fed. The farmer goes out to the barn and using a pitchfork, loads the stored hay onto his truck to take out to his cattle. As he does this, he often notices a thick yellow haze, composed of thermophilic actinomycetes bacteria, arising from the pile of hay. He does his job, goes home, has supper, and then wakes at midnight short of breath, often with a fever. He goes to the emergency room. The doctor does a chest radiograph, tells the farmer he has water on his lungs, and gives him a diuretic and in a few hours the farmer goes home. But the episode repeats every time he goes out to the barn to feed his cattle. Unless, the correct diagnosis is made, over time the farmer's lungs will become permanently scarred. This disease, of course, is called Farmer's lung and occurs in between 0.4% to 7% of farmers.

The disease can also be seen in people who handle birds, especially parrots, and in people who have hot tubs. In the latter case it is due to exposure to the Mycobacterium avium complex. Other, more unique causes include "humidifier lung" seen in office works, "swimming pool lung" seen in up to 37% of lifeguards, and "polyurethane foam lung" seen in up to 27% of workers at an injection molding plant.

The disease is caused by an intense immune reaction known as delayed hypersensitivity. The antigen or foreign invader sensitizes the cells of the respiratory tract which, when the cells are again exposed to the antigen, cause an immunologic reaction, resulting in granuloma formation.

The American Thoracic Society divides the disease into two groups, non-fibrotic or purely inflammatory, and fibrotic. Symptoms and signs are similar in both groups although the non-fibrotic group was more likely to have an acute episode or series of acute episodes, while the fibrotic group usually presented with an insidious and more indolent illness. The non-fibrotic group shows a ground glass infiltrate as well as tiny centrilobular nodules on HRCT while the fibrotic group shows changes of mid-lung traction bronchiectasis and honeycombing.

Clinically, the patient can present with an acute illness with shortness of breath, fever, and cough. More likely, the patient will be seen with chronic shortness of breath. In the acute case, the chest radiograph will look like pulmonary edema. In the chronic case, the chest x-ray will show interstitial fibrosis more pronounced in the upper part of the chest. A HRCAT scan will confirm these findings.

The diagnosis is based almost entirely on clinical suspicion. If the doctor does not suspect the disease, he will not diagnose it. A thorough work history is the key! The doctor must also ask about hobbies, such as woodworking, as well as their 8-5 job. If the doctor makes the diagnosis, the patient will do reasonably well; at least he will not get worse. If the doctor fails to make the diagnosis, the pulmonary fibrosis will worsen. The patient may die from his disease.

Confirmation of the diagnosis can be made by finding precipitating antibodies to the suspected antigen in the patient's blood. By itself, the test is not helpful. Almost all farmers will have precipitating antibodies to the thermophilic actinomycetes antigen, but only a handful will get Farmer's Lung. Skin testing, which depends on IgE antibodies, is not helpful.

The treatment is simply avoidance of the antigen though, if the patient is quite ill, corticosteroids may be used.

The Pneumoconiosis or Occupational Lung Diseases include Asbestosis and Silicosis. **Asbestosis** is caused by inhalation of the asbestos fiber. The fiber is very long and thin, shaped like a spear. When it is inhaled it impinges on the small airways and causes small airways disease. Macrophages rush to limit the damage the fiber causes, but they are unable to eliminate it. The fiber slowly works its way into the parenchyma of the lung causing more and more damage as it goes. The fiber may migrate all the way to the pleura. While some of the fibers are coughed out, at least 90% are retained and continue to cause increasing amounts of fibrosis over time.

Typically, the patient with asbestosis has a history of working with the fiber. He may have been an insulator in a refinery. He may have been a boilermaker applying insulation to a boiler. He may have been a roofer. He may have worked in an auto body repair shop with a compound called "Bondo." But, surprisingly most of the patients with severe disease, in my experience, have been painters who "taped and floated" a sealant called "Gold-Bond Sealant," which was made with asbestos, and electricians who worked alongside the insulators but never work masks. The disease can develop in anyone working with asbestos for more than 3 years. It will take, however, ten years for the symptoms to begin to appear.

Generally, the patient will present with cough and shortness of breath. Clubbing may occur. But if clubbing is present, be wary that the patient may have a cancer of the lung. The asbestos fiber also increases the risk of lung cancer! The chest radiograph and HRCAT scan will show a pattern that looks exactly like UIP, except that there may be pleural disease present. The pleural disease can be a pleural effusion or a calcified pleural plaque or may even be a cancer called a mesothelioma.

Pulmonary functions done early in the course of the disease may show an obstructive pattern involving the small airways, while patients who have had the disease for some time show a restrictive disease. The diffusing capacity is decreased.

The diagnosis is based solely on history. The diagnostic criteria are a history of exposure to the asbestos fiber, a latency period, the time from the onset of the patient's exposure to the fiber until the patient has symptoms, of ten years or more, and evidence of the disease such as shortness of breath, an abnormal chest radiograph, an abnormal HRCAT scan, or abnormal pulmonary function testing. A biopsy is generally not needed for the diagnosis.

Treatment is essentially symptomatic. Many patients will need oxygen and pulmonary rehabilitation.

One misconception is that asbestos is not allowed in the United States. That was not true until March 18 of 2024 when the Environmental Protection Agency finally banned the only form of asbestos that was currently imported into the United States. Only "white asbestos" which is used in brakes, as well as in making chlorine will be banned and the ban will take ten years to go into effect. The other five forms of asbestos, which are much more dangerous than "white asbestos" were not banned. The EPA was blocked from implementing a congressional ban in 2017 by President Trump who described it as "the greatest fire-proofing material ever made. Currently 50 countries have banned the material. More asbestos is mined now in the United States than in the early 1970's, but it is shipped to Africa and Asia. Thus, immigrants from these parts of the world who present with interstitial lung disease must be asked about their work history in detail.

The asbestos fiber can also cause all the different types of lung cancer as well as mesothelioma which is a cancer of the pleura.

Silicosis is caused by exposure to silica which is a small round particle made up of silicon dioxide. The disease is most often found in sandblasters, miners, tool-sharpeners, and toolmakers, who often use a quartz wheel for sharpening. It is the oldest of all the pneumoconiosis or occupational lung diseases. It was first described in gold miners of Eastern Europe in the 18th century. It was not unusual for a woman to go through several husbands all of whom were miners and all of whom died of silicosis after just a few years working in the mine. In one sense, the development of pulmonary function testing is due, at least in part, to silicosis. The owners of the mine, usually the rulers of the country, needed a way to determine if someone had significant disability from working in the mines. Thus, the need for pulmonary testing.

The silica particle is quite reactive. When it is inhaled, the macrophages engulf the silica, but the charged surface of the particle kills the macrophage. More and more macrophages arrive to cordon off the invader but all of them are killed resulting in fibrous, peribronchial granulomata. The granulomas grow in size, often becoming quite massive. Over time, generally about twenty or thirty years, the patient develops respiratory failure and dies.

Typically, the disease presents with shortness of breath. A chest x-ray will show numerous granulomata involving the upper lobes often associated with the presence of a large calcified hilar lymph node.

On rare occasions, acute silicosis may also occur. The Hawks Nest Tunnel disaster occurred in the early 1930's near the Gauley Bridge in West Virginia. It was part of a large hydroelectric project. About 500 or more men who were working at the tunnel died over a period of a few months. While supervisors at the project wore masks, the men working in the tunnel were not given any protective devices at all. When the men stopped writing home, some of their wives tried to get help from the government to find out what happened but the government refused. Some of them appealed to the New York Times for help. The newspaper sent reporters to the area and discovered the disaster. They found a mass grave. Many of the men died with acute silicosis, which resembles ARDS. Shortly after the discovery, Congress enacted legislation to prevent another such calamity.

Patients with silicosis are interesting because the disease is associated with autoimmune diseases such as rheumatoid arthritis. In addition, patients with silicosis may develop tuberculosis or become infected with the Mycobacterium avium complex bacteria.

There are many causes of occupational lung disease. Again, the patient's caretakers must always take a detailed work and hobby history.

Seminars in Respiratory Disease

Suggestions for minor papers

1. What is the six-minute walk?
2. What criteria are required to make a diagnosis of asbestosis?
3. Did Alfonse's parents have congestive heart failure or asbestosis?
4. What types of occupations are associated with asbestosis and silicosis?
5. What is 'taping and floating?"
6. What diseases are associated with clubbing of the fingers?

Peter A. Petroff, MD

Eight

Neurological Diseases

Neurological diseases can affect the lungs in two ways. The most obvious is by causing diaphragmatic and chest wall muscle weakness or paralysis leading directly to hypercarbic respiratory failure. Secondly, neurological diseases can affect the brainstem, the most primitive part of the brain, the part which controls our breathing and swallowing, resulting in chronic aspiration and subsequent pneumonia.

Some diseases affect the motor part of the cerebral cortex, the motor neurons, or the skeletal muscles, causing respiratory failure. A stroke or cerebrovascular accident (CVA) can paralyze one side of the body. Poliomyelitis, a disease of the anterior horn of the spinal cord, can cause loss of function of the diaphragm and all the muscles of the chest wall. Severe Myasthenia gravis (MG), due to disease of the neuromuscular junction, can impair the function of the chest wall muscles. Guillain-Barré (GB) or Ascending Paralysis, a disease which destroys the myelin sheath which provides nourishment for the neurons, can also cause total respiratory muscle paralysis. Diseases affecting the autonomic centers of the brainstem responsible for controlling the muscles of speech and swallowing will cause chronic aspiration. Most commonly this is due to multiple tiny strokes involving the brainstem which is called "pseudobulbar palsy." It can also be caused by a neurological condition such as Amyotrophic Lateral Sclerosis (ALS), a disease of the motor neurons of the lateral column of the spinal cord and the brainstem.

Treatment depends on the type of the disorder. If the disease causes respiratory muscle weakness, then ventilatory support either by non-invasive ventilation (NIV) or even mechanical ventilation is the key. If on the other hand, the problem is chronic aspiration then the treatment must be directed at either relearning how to swallow, if that is possible, or, if it is not possible, then nourishment must be provided by a feeding tube, usually a percutaneous endoscopic gastrostomy (PEG).

As of this moment there are very few neurological diseases which can be treated directly. For most of the common diseases supportive care while the patient heals, followed by physical therapy and rehabilitation are the most important aspects of care.

Peter A. Petroff, MD

Case Presentations

1.

Jane A. is a very pleasant 23-year-old senior at a nearby university. She returns to the emergency room with shortness of breath. She states she was in the emergency room two days before because she had tingling in her toes and fingers. The doctor who examined her said it was her "nerves." "I told him that I have an upcoming examination in a very difficult course." The doctor gave her a medicine to "calm her down."

Yesterday, she noticed that she had trouble getting out of a chair and the tingling had climbed up to her ankles. This morning she needed help walking. Now, she cannot even stand without help. She is especially concerned because she has had some choking episodes.

Jane's past history is largely unremarkable. She is an excellent student. She is studying to be a respiratory therapist. Some of her courses involve direct hospital care, of course, and three weeks ago, she was exposed to a child who had Campylobacter gastroenteritis. The little girl was quite ill for almost two weeks but finally pulled through.

Jane is a never smoker. She does not drink or use recreational drugs of any kind. She does not take any medications and has no drug allergies. She has never had surgery, nor has she ever been hospitalized. Her mother had asthma and that is why she wanted to become a respiratory therapist.

Her examination reveals her to be quite weak and the weakness involves all her extremities. In addition, she has difficulty raising her head off the pillow. Her blood pressure, pulse rate and SaO2 are all normal. Her head and neck examination are also unremarkable. Her lungs are clear though the breath sounds are markedly decreased. The abdominal exam is unremarkable though muscle tone is diminished. She has a near-complete flaccid paralysis of her legs with absent patellar reflexes.

At this point, the doctor is reasonably sure of Jane's diagnosis. He obtains routine laboratory which he feels will serve as a baseline. He also orders a portable chest radiograph and arterial blood gases. Most importantly, he immediately asks the respiratory therapist stationed in the emergency room to do a bedside vital capacity and determine the patient's maximum inspiratory pressure.

The complete blood count and chemistry profile are normal as was a urinalysis. Serologic studies for Campylobacter are still pending. The chest radiograph shows decreased lung volumes but no definite infiltrates. The blood gases on room air are as follows: paO2 72, pCO2 40, pH 7.38, HCO3 24. The vital capacity is 1.6 liters, and the peak inspiratory pressure is 20.

The doctor calculated the A-a O2 gradient, "A is the atmospheric pressure minus 1.25 times the pCO2 or 150 – 50 is 100. The little "a" is the arterial pO2 which is 72. Hence the A-a O2 gradient is 100 minus 72 or 28 which is abnormally high for a woman in her early 20's."

The emergency room physician calls the admitting intensivist and the neurologist on call. The patient must be admitted to the ICU. She is begun on intravenous immunoglobulin or "IV-IG" and oxygen. Bedside vital capacities and maximum inspiratory pressures are to be done every two hours. A nasogastric (NG) feeding tube is placed. She is also begun on subcutaneous Lovenox (low molecular weight heparin) and Protonix given via her NG tube.

Over the next six hours the vital capacity falls from 1.6 liters to .8 liters. The respiratory rate increases to 26 breaths a minute. The intensivist intubates the patient with a 7 ET tube and places her on a volume-controlled ventilator with the following settings: AC of 12, TV 420 cc, 40% O2 and PEEP of 5 cm H2O. Her blood gases are as follows: pO2 of 145, pCO2 of 42, pH of 7.40 and HCO3 of 24. He decreased her O2 to 30%.

The following day, a gastroenterologist removes the feeding tube and inserts a PEG tube. The ventilatory settings and medications remain unchanged. Over the next several days her condition waxes and wanes. The paralysis becomes quite severe. Her eyes are taped closed to prevent drying of her corneas. She is placed on a special bed and mattress to prevent decubiti from developing. Her blood pressure and pulse rate fluctuate wildly; a cardiologist is called to help manage the autonomic dysfunction. She is kept sedated though not paralyzed.

After nearly three weeks of care, the paralysis begins to wane. Jane can open and close her eyes and lift her head off the pillow without assistance. She can even move her legs and lift her arms a little. Her spontaneous vital capacity increased from 0.4 liters to 1.2 liters. She is placed on a T-piece for a half hour. Her blood gases on the T piece are: pO2 of 108, pCO2 of 36, pH of 7.46, HCO3 of 24. The intensivist extubates her and places her on a 40% Ventimask. Over the next 24 hours her vital capacity increases to 2 liters. She is transferred out of the ICU and intensive physical therapy is begun. After another week, she is transferred to a rehabilitation hospital.

2.

Suzette T., a 35-year-old woman, came to the neurology clinic because of problems with her eyes. She told the neurologist she works as a television newscaster. Last week one of her viewers watching her on television texted the station that he was concerned she had a problem with her eyes. "The text said that I crossed my eyes after a few seconds after I began to read the news on the teleprompter. I was not even aware of it. Then I stared at a mirror and sure enough my eyes crossed, and for an instant I had double vision."

Suzette went on, "I've also noticed that my eyelids droop and sometimes my speech isn't as clear as it ought to be."

She had no other history of neurologic disease although she said that sometimes, "water goes down the wrong pipe."

She was a never-smoker. She drank occasionally. She did not take any medications and had no drug allergies. She had no history of surgery or medical admissions.

Her BP was 124/72; her pulse was 62; her O2 saturation was 96%. She was 5'4" tall and weighed 104 lbs.

The doctor asked her to stare at a chart that hung on the wall. After just a few seconds her left eye deviated towards the right and the right eyelid drooped a third of the way down over the eye, as if she were winking.

He told her to keep staring at the chart. He got some ice from the office refrigerator and poured it into a surgical glove. He then placed the gloved ice gently over her right eye. In a few moments, the "droop" had nearly completely resolved.

The doctor did a thorough physical examination which was totally normal.

"Suzette, I believe you have Myasthenia gravis, a type of nerve disease. I need to get some studies to confirm it including some blood tests, a CAT scan of your chest to look at your thymus gland, and an electrical test to confirm the diagnosis."

The blood tests showed antibodies against the acetylcholine receptor but not against a receptor-associated-protein called "muscle specific tyrosine kinase." The CAT scan of the chest showed that the thymus gland was enlarged. The electrodiagnostic testing showed that with repetitive nerve stimulation Suzette's muscle contraction (action potential) weakened. The technician also did a single fiber electromyography. A single nerve that supplied two separate muscle fibers was identified. Normally when the nerve signals the muscles both will fire at the same time. However, patients with myasthenia gravis will have variability or "jitter" in the muscle response. One will fire before the other. Suzette's test confirmed increased "jitter." Blood tests done to detect autoimmune diseases including thyroid disease were negative.

Suzette returned to the doctor's office a week later. The doctor told her that the tests confirmed the diagnosis of Myasthenia. He advised her to become extremely cautious about any medication, even over the counter medications, "Take only the medications you absolutely need." He also gave her a list of medicines which aggravate myasthenia or can precipitate a crisis.

He went on, "All sedating drugs must be avoided, even Benadryl. In addition, antibiotics such as Levaquin, Cipro, aminoglycosides, and one called telithromycin must be avoided. Even magnesium sulfate, which some people take for muscle cramps, can cause Myasthenia to worsen abruptly. Heart medicines like B blockers and even medicines to lower the cholesterol level have to be used very carefully."

He then prescribed Mestinon or pyridostigmine, 30 mg three times a day with meals, gradually increasing the dose to 90 mg four times a day. He told her to back down on the dose if she gets diarrhea or cramping in her stomach. He also told her that if the dose is too high, she could get weakness that looks just like her myasthenia.

Suzette did well for the next year and a half. She had no more texts from viewers about her double vision and was working full-time. Then, she got pregnant. She began noticing a recurrence of her double vision. In addition, she developed frequent choking episodes and muscle weakness.

Sometimes she had a hard time even lifting her head off the pillow. The weakness worsened over just a few days. She was brought to the emergency room by her husband because of a severe cough.

In the ER, the doctor noted that she had a fever, cough with phlegm, and profound weakness. The cough was productive of rust colored phlegm. Her examination confirmed inspiratory crackles over the right lower lobe. Of more concern her vital capacity was only 1.6 liters. The doctor admitted her to the ICU under the care of the hospital intensivist.

The intensivist ordered a blood count, blood cultures, ABGs and a chest radiograph. He began her on Penicillin IV (intravenous) as well as IV fluids. He made her NPO (nothing by mouth). He also began her on a course of IV-IG as well as high dose IV corticosteroids. Her vital capacity was only 1.2 liters on arrival in the ICU and the intensivist chose, with her consent, to intubate her and begin her on mechanical ventilation. The settings were: assist control of 16 with a TV of 400 cc, 40% oxygen and 5 cm PEEP. An NG tube was placed, and intermittent compressive stockings were used to prevent the development of clots.

The blood count showed a white cell count of 16,400. The chest radiograph showed a right lower lobe pneumonia. The blood cultures were still pending. The ABGs were done after intubation. The pO2 was 115, the pCO2 was 32, the pH was 7.48, and the HCO3 was 24. The ventilator rate was decreased to 14 and the fiO2 to 35%.

Over the next week the patient improved. Her temperature returned to normal, and the secretions diminished. By the seventh day post intubation her vital capacity was 1.6 liters. The Mestinon was restarted via the NG tube and the dose of steroids slowly decreased. On the ninth day, she was extubated following a successful trial of spontaneous breathing.

She was discharged on low dose prednisone as well as her Mestinon. The remainder of her pregnancy was uneventful, and she delivered a healthy little girl.

3.

Foster C. comes to the clinic because of "funny twitching in my muscles." He is a 65-year-old male, retired electrician, who worked at a large chemical plant in Houston. He states that he first noticed the twitching about six months before. He says, "Sometimes my biceps twitch; sometimes it's the muscles in my thigh. It can be anywhere." He also has noticed that he is weaker. He used to walk a mile every day but had to give it up.

The doctor asks about swallowing and choking. Foster says that he has had more problems with swallowing, especially liquids. He has also lost about ten lbs. over the last six months, "Without even trying." He quickly adds, "I needed to lose it anyway." He has not had any pain, double vision, or any changes in sensation such as an abnormal feeling or taste or smell.

He has been healthy otherwise. He smokes about a half a pack of cigarettes a day and drinks one or two beers every day. He takes Norvasc for his blood pressure. He is allergic to penicillin. He had an appendectomy when he was twenty but has otherwise never been in the hospital. His family history is non-contributory. No one in the family ever had any nerve problems.

His BP is 148/94; his pulse is 78; his O2 saturation is 92%. He is 5'10" tall and weighs 175 lbs.

His examination is unremarkable except for marked symmetrically decreased breath sounds without any adventitious sounds and the presence of intermittent muscular fasciculations and markedly hyperactive tendon reflexes. He is unable to stand from a sitting position in a chair without assistance.

The doctor orders routine blood tests including a CBC, chemistry panel, an autoimmune panel, a creatine kinase, and a urinalysis. Because of history of smoking, he also orders a chest radiograph. Lastly, he sends Foster for electrodiagnostic testing, MRI of his brain, and a spinal tap.

The electrodiagnostic testing confirms the presence of fasciculations as well as other changes consistent with Amyotrophic Lateral Sclerosis. The MRI of his brain is normal. The creatine kinase is markedly elevated (over 1000 units/liter). The spinal tap shows a normal cell count and protein level.

The patient returns after the study results come back. The doctor tells him that he likely has Amyotrophic Lateral Sclerosis but "only time would tell for sure if the diagnosis is correct." The doctor explains what to expect and about some new medications that slow the progression of the disease as well as experimental therapy under development including gene therapy. He also schedules pulmonary function testing which shows a vital capacity of 55% of predicted.

Foster agrees to start Riluzole, 50 mg, twice a day. Over the next two years, the patient's condition deteriorates. He has more and more shortness of breath and becomes weaker and weaker. The vital capacity gradually falls to 1.2 liters. Finally, he is wheelchair dependent. Aspiration is a constant threat. The patient complains about severe morning headaches. His O2 saturation in the doctor's office is 88%. After discussion with the patient, the doctor begins Foster on Non-Invasive Ventilation (NIV) at night as well as the use of "sip" ventilation during the day. A PEG tube is placed in order to provide nutrition.

Over the next few months, Foster becomes bedbound and requires NIV around the clock. The doctor makes home visits to follow his patient who can no longer come to the office. On the last visit, the doctor and Foster discuss additional therapy. Does Foster want to have a tracheostomy and long-term mechanical ventilation? It would mean that Foster would have to go to a nursing home.

Without hesitation, Foster says no. He would rather die at home. He is begun on Hospice Care and dies two weeks later.

Background for the presentations

The first patient has a neurologic disorder called Guillain-Barré. She had a prior history of an exposure to an infectious disease known to cause the disorder followed by a symmetrical neurological condition involving both his sensory and motor neurons in an ascending pattern. Over a period of just a few days, she became paralyzed and ventilatory dependent but within just three weeks her neurological condition nearly completely resolved. The second patient has Myasthenia gravis which began as ocular myasthenia and was well controlled on Mestinon alone. However, when she became pregnant, she experienced a Myasthenic Crisis and had to be intubated and ventilated. Nevertheless, with IVIG, steroids, and excellent supportive care she did well and went on to a full recovery. The last patient has Amyotrophic Lateral Sclerosis which presented as diffuse muscle weakness, hyperreflexia and fasciculations, findings consistent with combined upper and lower motor neuron disease. His course was downhill from the start as it always is with this condition, and he chose not to have invasive mechanical ventilation.

Important points

1. A Myasthenic crisis can be precipitated by infection, pregnancy, childbirth, or surgery. It can also occur spontaneously.
2. About 10% of patients with Myasthenia will have a Myasthenic crisis at least once in the course of their disease.
3. About 30% of patients with Guillain-Barré will need to be intubated. NIV is a second option.
4. Plasmapheresis and IVIG are equally effective in treating both Guillain-Barré and the Myasthenic crisis.
5. The patient with ALS must be allowed to choose how he or she will be treated. It is not our decision. We must always be truthful with our patients. They have a right to know even if the outcome is likely to be bad.
6. ALS and Myasthenia gravis involve only the motor neurons while Guillain-Barré involves both the myelinated motor and sensory fibers.
7. One hallmark of ALS is the exaggerated emotional response. They can start laughing or crying for little reason. This is believed to be due to the disease involving the brainstem and is called "pseudobulbar affect."

Discussion

The nervous system is a highly integrated complex organ. It allows us to interact with and even change our environment. It has a sensory arm which transmits signals from our skin, eyes, ears, and taste buds to the appropriate section of our brain where the signals are first recognized then integrated so that the appropriate response can be sent down motor neurons from our brain to the muscles of our legs or arms.

Some of the nerve fibers are wrapped in myelin. These nerves conduct impulses faster because the electrical excitation jumps from one Node of Ranvier to the next rather than slowly making its way along the nerve. In addition, there are many types of sensations such as touch, pain, and vibration, light, color, sound, and smell. Different types of fibers carry the different signals. Touch sensation is carried in myelinated fibers, so the conduction is fast, while most pain fibers are unmyelinated and are therefore slow conducting. However, some of the pain fibers, especially those related to a burning sensation, are myelinated and fast conducting. Sensory fibers enter the dorsal ganglion just outside the spinal cord which functions like a railway station, allowing the peripheral nerves to connect with the central sensory nerves which then enter the spinal cord at the dorsal horn and travel up the spinal tract in the anterolateral spinal tract and ascend to the sensory portion (the parietal area) of the brain.

The motor fibers, which are all myelinated, descend from the temporal portion of the cerebral cortex and then cross just below the medulla. Thus, the right side of the brain controls the left arm and left leg and vice versa. These upper motor neuron fibers communicate with lower motor neurons in the anterior horn of the spinal cord. The lower motor neurons then communicate with muscle cells at the neuromuscular junction.

A disease can affect any portion of the system. A stroke or cerebrovascular accident causes direct damage to the brain. In addition, there are diseases that involve the upper motor neurons such as Amyotrophic Lateral Sclerosis, diseases that involve the anterior horn of the spinal cord such as Poliomyelitis, diseases that involve the lower motor neurons such as Guillain-Barre, diseases that involve the junction between the neurons and muscle cells such as Myasthenia Gravis, as well as diseases which involve the muscles themselves such as Myositis. Adding even more complexity, if the upper motor neurons are damaged, the lower motor neurons with which they interact will also die and if the lower motor neurons die, the muscles they innervate will die as well.

In addition to the motor and sensory nerves, there are fibers which are not under our direct control. This part of the nervous system is called the autonomic nervous system. This system is important in breathing, swallowing, digesting our food, maintaining our balance, controlling our heart rate, controlling our blood pressure, and many other functions too numerous to list. There are even diseases that affect only the autonomic nervous system. The nerve fibers of the autonomic system are not covered with a myelin sheath.

In this section we want to deal with four diseases of the nervous system, each completely different with a different etiology and different pathological and clinical picture, but all of which can affect the lung indirectly. While these diseases are not common, they are most certainly not rare. The respiratory therapist will encounter these diseases on a regular basis.

Guillain-Barré is an autoimmune disease causing an acute but reversible polyradiculoneuropathy (a disease affecting many peripheral nerves which originate at the level of the nerve roots). There are between 5000 and 6000 new cases every year. The disease most often affects young adults. Men are more likely to get the disease than women.

Most often, the disease is preceded by an infectious disease, most commonly gastroenteritis caused by Campylobacter jejuni. Other infections included Covid-19, Herpes virus infection, HIV infection, and Mycoplasma pneumoniae infection. An influenza vaccination may also cause the disorder. The yearly flu vaccine causes one case per million vaccinations. The swine flu vaccine in 1976 caused about 8 cases of Guillain-Barré per million vaccinations, about 8 times more than normal.

The disease is an autoimmune disease. The vaccine or infection causes the production of antibodies which not only attack the infectious agent but also attack the nerve roots which results in damage to the myelin sheath as well as the axon of the nerve. The myelin sheath is important. It wraps around the axon of the nerves speeding conduction as well as providing nutrition for the axon. Normally, nerve conduction is caused by serial depolarization of the action potential. The myelin sheath allows the depolarization to jump from one Node of Ranvier to the next.

Typically, the disease begins in the longest nerves, the nerves to the legs, with symptoms of numbness and weakness. Over a period of just a few days, the weakness and numbness ascend to involve the arms and then, in some patients, the head and neck. The cranial nerves may be involved resulting in dysphagia and aspiration. The autonomic system is involved in more than a third of patients resulting in bowel dysfunction, labile blood pressure, and significant cardiac arrhythmias. The patient often has severe neck and back pain.

Examination confirms the weakness and sensory loss. A key finding is that the deep tendon reflexes are decreased to absent. Examination of the cerebrospinal fluid shows an elevated protein with a normal white cell count in 2/3rds of patients. This is called "albumin-cytologic dissociation" and is a hallmark of the disease.

The diagnosis of Guillain-Barré is based on the clinical presentation of progressive (several days to four weeks) **and** symmetrical muscle weakness associated with absent or decreased deep tendon reflexes, supported by the findings of the cerebrospinal fluid and characteristic electrodiagnostic testing.

The disease generally peaks at 3 to 4 weeks. Then the patient begins to improve as remyelination begins. Immunotherapeutic treatment consists of either a course of high dose intravenous IVIG or serial plasma-pheresis. Both therapies are equally effective and there is no evidence that using both therapies is any better than just using one of the two therapies. The IVIG is pooled gamma globulin. Its mechanism of action is unknown but likely relates to downregulating the inflammatory response causing the destruction of myelin. Plasmapheresis or plasma exchange likely removes the antibodies which cause the disease. Immunotherapy must begin within four weeks of onset of the illness. IVIG is given at 0.4 g/kg per day for five days. The patient is also pretreated with Tylenol and diphenhydramine. Side effects include low blood pressure, nausea, headache, and rash. Even kidney failure may occur.

Corticosteroids have never been shown to be helpful and should be avoided.

Supportive care is most important. Almost all patients with Guillain-Barré need to be hospitalized and most of these patients will be best treated in the ICU. 30% of the patients will require mechanical ventilation for at least some time. In addition to respiratory failure and the constant threat of aspiration, autonomic instability is a major problem in 70% of patients. Thus, the patients require intense monitoring of their cardiac and respiratory parameters including telemetry, automatic blood pressure monitoring, and frequent checks of their vital capacity. They all require therapy to prevent clots, usually Lovenox or low molecular weight heparin. Frequent turning of the patient or a Rotobed is used to prevent decubiti. Nutritional support is also extremely important.

There are several indications[4] for intubation of the patient:

1. Shortness of breath while speaking or at rest
2. Patients who are using accessory muscles to breath
3. Those patients who can't count to 15 in one breath
4. Patients who have a respiratory rate more than 30 breaths/minute, an oxygen saturation of less than 92% on oxygen, a FVC < 20 ml/kg, an MEP less than 40 cm H2O, or acute hypercapnia
5. Those patients with impaired swallowing or who are unable to clear their secretions.

Patients with Guillain-Barré often have severe neck and lumbar pain requiring medical therapy. Medications used for pain include non-steroidal anti-inflammatory medications, epidural morphine sulfate, and Gabapentin.

Physical therapy, occupational therapy, and speech therapy become the mainstay of treatment in the patient recovering from Guillain-Barré. They should be started as soon as possible.

Older patients, patients with a rapid onset of disease and patients with severe weakness on admission to hospital have a much worse prognosis. Most patients will do well but about 5% will die of the disease. If the patient requires mechanical ventilation the mortality rate is 20%. Within twelve months, 60% will have full recovery but 14% will still have severe motor problems.

Amyotrophic Lateral Sclerosis is the most common fatal neurodegenerative disease. It involves **both** the upper and lower motor neurons. The upper motor neurons run from the cerebral cortex to the anterior horn of the spinal cord and the lower motor neurons run the anterior horn to

---

[4] Suraj Ashok Muley MN, UpToDate, May 2, 2023

the neuromuscular junction. The involved nerves shrink and a pigmented lipid, normally seen with old age, accumulates inside the cells and cellular neurofilaments inclusions and Bunina bodies become more prominent. With the death of the lower motor neurons, the muscles they innervate atrophy. Hence the term "amyotrophic." As the nerves in the lateral columns of the spinal cord shrink and become stiff, that portion of the spinal cord feels hard or sclerotic.

The disease affects men more than women. The disorder becomes more and more common with advancing age beginning at about the age of fifty. About 2 people per 100,000 will get the disease in any year. In other words, there will be about 7,000 new cases in the United States every year. Smokers, people with exposure to pesticides and insecticides and people with military service appear to be at increased risk of getting the disease. The incidence of ALS is higher among veterans of the Gulf War. Ten percent of the cases are familial and inherited in an autosomal dominant pattern. But to date more than 20 causative genes have been identified. Multiple chromosomes appear to be involved. Many physicians now believe that ALS is a degenerative disease of aging similar to Alzheimer's disease but involving the neuromuscular system and not memory.

Symptoms of the disease include <u>asymmetrical</u> muscle weakness associated with atrophy of the muscles, morning muscle cramps which generally are precipitated by stretching, fasciculations or intermittent spontaneous muscle twitching that looks like worms crawling about under the skin, markedly increased deep tendon reflexes as well as difficulty swallowing, speaking, and chewing when the bulbar muscles become involved. Many patients will also have exaggerated emotional expressions with spontaneous crying and laughter for no reason at all. Most patients have little or no mental impairment. However, some patients, especially those with familial ALS have frontotemporal dementia which is characterized by problems with executive function and language. But memory is not a problem as it is with Alzheimer's disease.

The treatment of the disease is largely supportive. Two medications are currently available, both of which have shown minimal but definite slowing of the disease process. The first, Riluzole, diminishes glutamate release and prolongs survival. In one study the survival of patients at one year was increased from 58% to 74%. If the patient primarily had brainstem disease ("bulbar"), the one-year survival increased from 35% to 73%. The studies have been confirmed in "real life" studies. The medication is given by mouth twice a day. The most significant side effects include gastrointestinal symptoms as well as abnormal liver function tests. Edaravone is an antioxidant, a free-radical scavenger, that is believed to reduce oxidative stress. It is given either intravenously or orally for ten to fourteen days on the fourteen days off. The drug was approved by the FDA in 2017, and in at least one study showed the agent slowed progression by 33% in patients only when the drug was begun early in the course of the illness. The most serious side effect of Edaravone is asthma since the drug contains sulfites and 5% of asthmatics develop asthma when exposed to sodium bisulfite. Sodium phenylbutyrate-Taurursodiol was approved by the FDA in 2022. The drug reduces neuronal cell death and has been shown to slow progression of ALS. The drug is taken orally. All three agents can be used together.

Several types of medication are in development including medicines to activate muscles and medicines to altar gene expression. An excellent discussion of upcoming medications and even some old medication worthy of being reevaluated including high dose vitamin B12 can be found in up UpToDate issue dated May 9, 2023, and current through Jan 24. The article was authored by Namita Goyal, MD, Nestor Galvez-Jimenez Md, and Merit Cudkowicz MD.

Supportive care is paramount. Non-invasive ventilation (NIV) and "sip" ventilation can be utilized to assist the patient's respiratory status. A "Cough Assist Device" is useful to help the patient clear secretions. A gastrostomy can be used to provide nutrition. In addition, there are several devices that will help make the patient's speech more intelligible. Physical therapy and, especially, occupational therapy are important as well.

Some patients will choose to live with a tracheostomy and ventilator. Some will not. The life expectancy for a patient with ALS is 4 years on average. However about 10 to 20% will survive for more than ten years. The two most famous people who died of ALS are Steven Hawking and Lou Gehrig.

Myasthenia gravis is an autoimmune disease which affects the neuromuscular junction, the site where the nerve innervates and activates the muscle. The disease causes muscle weakness which worsens with repetitive use of the muscle.

The nerve ending contains vesicles or tiny globules filled with molecules of acetyl choline. When the nerve is activated, the action potential flows down the nerve to the nerve ending causing the release of these vesicles into the space between the nerve and the muscle. The vesicles release their acetyl choline which migrates to the surface of the muscle fiber which has innumerable receptors for the acetyl choline. The acetyl choline binds to the receptor deforming the cell surface and causing the rapid flow of sodium into the muscle fiber setting off the muscle's action potential. The action potential flows along the muscle fiber causing the release of intracellular calcium which triggers the reaction between actin and myosin resulting in muscle contraction.

Most patients with myasthenia gravis have antibodies directed at the acetyl choline receptors. The antibodies reduce the number of receptor sites and deform the surface of the muscle fiber. The antibodies may form because muscle-like cells in the Thymus gland, called myoid cells, are seen as foreign antigens. The antibodies attack both the myoid cells and the acetyl choline receptors.

The disease affects women more often than men but interestingly women are generally affected in their twenties and thirties and men in their fifties and sixties. The disease also has striking geographic distributions. It is common in the Mediterranean parts of Europe while much less common in northern Europe. In Asia, Myasthenia occurs in children and young adults half of the time, but childhood disease is distinctly unusual in America and Europe.

The hallmark clinical features are weakness associated with <u>fatigability</u>. The weakness worsens with repetitive use. Unlike Guillain-Barré which generally begins in the feet and moves upward, Myasthenia begins in the head and moves downward. The earliest symptoms of Myasthenia generally involve the eyes with ptosis (the upper lids drift downwards) and oculomotor (eye muscle) weakness causing double vision. Involvement of the muscles of the face causes a grimace or snarl when the patient attempts to smile. Speech may be "mushy" due to weakness of the tongue or "nasal" due to weakness of the palate. Chewing meat can really be a problem especially about half-way through the meal. Nasal regurgitation of liquids may occur as well. Unlike Guillain-Barré, Myasthenia involves the proximal muscles of the arm and leg. The deep tendon reflexes are normal.

The diagnosis of myasthenia can be made at the bedside if the patient has ptosis by using the ice-pact test. An ice pack is placed over the involved eye and the degree of ptosis is observed. If there is a significant response the diagnosis is established. Most patients today are diagnosed by finding antibodies to either the **acetyl choline receptor** or to **muscle-specific tyrosine kinase**. The antibody to the acetyl choline receptor is 85% sensitive except in patients who have only ocular myasthenia where it is only about 50% sensitive. The type of antibody also distinguishes between the two types of myasthenia. Typical myasthenia (90% of all myasthenia patients) is characterized by antibodies to the acetyl choline receptor. Generally, these patient presents with ptosis and double vision. Patients with the much less common disorder characterized by the presence of antibodies to tyrosine kinase (1 to 10% of patients with myasthenia) tend to be younger and to be female. Ptosis and double vision are much less commonly seen. However, there is more proximal muscle weakness as well as weakness of the chest wall and abdomen, facial weakness, and respiratory distress. **In fact, 60% of patients with antibodies to tyrosine kinase have respiratory distress**.

In the past edrophonium testing was done routinely to make the diagnosis. The chemical is no longer available in the United States. Edrophonium is a quick acting anticholinesterase inhibitor with a short duration of activity (less than ten minutes). It blocks the breakdown of acetyl choline increasing the amount of acetyl choline at the neuromuscular junction and enhancing the excitation of the muscle cells. The drug can cause severe side effects including syncope, bradycardia, or even asthma, so atropine must be at hand when the test is done. Because of the risks associated with edrophonium today it is used only if all other diagnostic tests fail to make the diagnosis in a patient that likely has Myasthenia.

Electrodiagnostic testing can be done to confirm the diagnosis. In the patient with myasthenia, repetitive nerve stimulation causes the muscle fibers to show progressively reduced action potential. In addition, single nerve fiber testing is often helpful. A nerve fiber is chosen which innervates two muscle fibers. The nerve fiber is stimulated and the action potential from each muscle fiber is observed. Normally the muscle fibers are activated at the same time but with myasthenia there is variability between the times for muscle fiber activation which is called "jitter." This test is positive in 90% of patients with myasthenia. However, the test is not specific. It can be positive in Guillain-Barré Syndrome, motor neuron disease, polymyositis, and peripheral neuropathies.

All patients with myasthenia gravis should have pulmonary function testing which will show a restrictive defect with normal diffusion. The pulmonary testing also establishes a baseline which can be used as a guide to the effectiveness of therapy.

The treatment of myasthenia involves the use of an anticholinesterase inhibitor, most commonly a medication called Mestinon or Pyridostigmine. The medication is begun at low doses three times a day and titrated up to the most effective dose. Too much Mestinon can cause "muscarinic side effects" such as nausea, diarrhea, and drooling. It can also cause weakness which mimics myasthenia. Patients with the tyrosine kinase antibodies do not do as well with Mestinon. For these patients, steroids and rituximab are more effective.

All patients with myasthenia should be considered for thymectomy or the removal of the thymus gland even if they do not have a Thymoma or tumor of the thymus. There is now extensive evidence of the clinical benefit of the surgery.

The mainstay of therapy has become the use of immunosuppressive agents. These include IV-IG, plasmapheresis, glucocorticoids, and drugs such as cyclosporine (used in transplant patients to prevent rejection), azathioprine (an anticancer agent), mycophenolate (a purine synthesis inhibitor) and rituximab or Rituxan (a monoclonal antibody which binds to B lymphocytes).

IV-IG and plasmapheresis are used to obtain immediate improvement in a Myasthenic crisis. Glucocorticoids and cyclosporine on the other hand require weeks to months to become effective while azathioprine and mycophenolate may require up to a year to see its maximum benefits.

While glucocorticoids have been shown to be very effective, there is a significant risk of a transient worsening when high does steroids are first begun. 10% of patients who begin high dose steroids will require intubation! The decline in function occurs between day 5 and 10 after starting the medication and lasts up to 5 days. Because of this steroids should always be begun in the hospital setting. The steroids should be tapered very slowly over several months to a maintenance dose of about 10 mg a day of prednisone.

Patients who are **acetyl choline receptor positive or seronegative** respond equally well to either azathioprine or mycophenolate mofetil. Both are "steroid sparing" agents. Patient who are **muscle-specific tyrosine kinase positive** are very likely to require continued steroid therapy although many respond to rituximab. Rituximab is a monoclonal antibody directed against the B cell membrane marker CD20. While it was first used against B cell lymphomas, it turns out that Myasthenia is also a B cell mediated disease. At the present time there are more than a half dozen additional antibody medications available to treat Myasthenia.

The Myasthenic Crisis is an acute exacerbation of Myasthenia characterized by profound weakness and usually respiratory failure. It is most often caused by an infection but both pregnancy and childbirth can be causes. In addition, certain medications including Cipro, Levaquin, Erythromycin, Zithromycin, Procainamide, Quinidine, and magnesium have been linked to the Myasthenic crisis. It is treated in the ICU with mechanical ventilation as well as the use of either IV-IG or plasmapheresis.

The prognosis of Myasthenia is improving steadily. At present the mortality rate is about 1.5%. More than 25% of patients obtain a sustained remission of their disease after immunosuppressive therapy and thymectomy. It is hard to imagine that a hundred years ago the mortality rate was 70%.

Multiple Sclerosis (MS) is the most common demyelinating disease of the central nervous system. It is the most frequent cause of permanent disability in young adults. Twice as many young women as young men are affected by the disease process. The disease most commonly affects people from their mid-teens to their thirties. The disease is likely autoimmune in causation and illnesses such as autoimmune diseases like systemic lupus erythematosus and thyroid disease are more common in patients with MS. There may be a genetic component as well. Monozygotic twins are more likely to share the disease than non-twin siblings. The risk for monozygotic twins is 20% while it is only 3-5% among siblings.

Environmental factors may also play a role, especially infection with the Epstein-Barr virus (EBV). The risk of MS doubles after an infection with this organism. Studies from throughout the world have shown that MS is more common in cold climates including Canada, Northern Europe, and the northern parts of the United States. The highest incidence of MS is in the Orkney Islands which are north of Scotland. In the tropics the incidence is up to twenty times less. At first the association with cold climate was felt to be due to race but subsequent studies show that Blacks in cold regions of the world are much more likely to get the disease than Blacks in warmer regions. Some scientists have attributed the geographical distribution to the effect of the sun on Vitamin D activation.

Overall, in the USA there are about 350,000 people who live with MS.

The pathological features of MS are characterized by the presence of "focal demyelinated plaques" associated with inflammatory changes located throughout the central nervous system. The most common sites of involvement are the optic nerve (optic neuritis), brainstem, spinal cord, cerebellum, and the white, and to lesser extent the gray matter of the brain.

The typical patient with MS has a progressive, but relapsing course of the disease though there is considerable variation. The disease will generally wax and wane with sudden episodes of worsening which may just as quickly improve, at least somewhat. However, over time, generally years, there will be more and more disability. But the disease can have a steady downhill course, or it may wax and wane with near complete recovery. A single lesion may occur without any recurrence or progression. Thus, the disease is highly variable. Most patients have an exacerbation about once every two years though the frequency, like much of MS, is quite variable. Life expectancy of the patient with MS is reduced by about 10 years. Thus, if the normal life expectancy is 84 years for the average woman, the woman with MS will live to about 74. The main causes of death are infection, respiratory disease, suicide, and cardiovascular disease.

Often the disease will present with sudden unilateral blindness. Other presentations include acute motor weakness, abnormal sensations, "electric-shock-like" sensations running down the back when the neck is flexed, dizziness, bladder disorders, and pain.

There are no specific clinical features that allow for a diagnosis of MS. Rather it is the totality of the presentation that matters. Typically, the patient is a young adult. There is a history of one or more neurological complaints with different neuroanatomic features over the preceding months. These changes will appear over hours to days and remit over weeks to months. The key to making the diagnosis is the MRI of the brain. If there are characteristic plaques **in locations of the brain that match the observed clinical features** the diagnosis is assured. The sensitivity of the MRI is 87% with a specificity of 73%.

If the MRI is not diagnostic then a spinal tap (lumbar puncture) should be done and the cerebrospinal fluid (CSF) studied, looking for "CSF-specific oligoclonal immunoglobulin G (IgG) bands" which are found in up to 95% of patients with definite MS. The CSF may also show increased lymphocytes, but the protein levels are generally normal. The presence of the immunoglobulin bands by themselves can be found in up to 8% of normal individuals.

Another test often used to confirm MS is the use of evoked potentials. In patients with MS, peripheral stimulation of a non-diseased area can result in characteristic electrical events in the central nervous system. Lastly, there are several autoantibodies which can be looked for.

Many other neurological diseases can mimic MS including encephalomyelitis (inflammation of the brain), Behçet disease, paraneoplastic disorders, polyarteritis nodosa, Sjogren's' syndrome, Sarcoidosis, neurosyphilis, B12 deficiency, Arnold-Chiari malformation, and systemic lupus erythematosus. Generally, time, the MRI, and the CSF studies will allow the correct diagnosis to be made.

Treatment is with the use of immune-modulating agents. These agents are used mainly for acute exacerbations. Their use in the long-term treatment of MS is limited because they can only be used for a few months or a year or two at most. Therefore, the cornerstone of therapy is largely supportive care including speech therapy, physical therapy, occupational therapy, and respiratory therapy.

Immune-modulating therapies include corticosteroids, Interferon Beta, cyclophosphamide, azathioprine, cladribine, cyclosporine, methotrexate, and human anti-CD20 monoclonal antibody *ocrelizumab*. Surprisingly, neither IV-IG nor plasma exchange have been shown to be effective. Early studies suggest stem cell transplantation may be helpful.

Ocrelizumab is one of the most effective therapies for MS. It is a monoclonal antibody directed against the CD20 molecule on mature B cells. Because it attacks mature B cells and not the developing or maturing B cells, both humeral immunity as well as the capacity to make new B cells is not interfered with. The agent reduces yearly relapses by 47% and decreases new CNS lesions by 95%. It is given by IV injection every six months. There is a downside to Ocrelizumab. Infusion reactions and lung infections including pneumonia may occur. The medication also nearly triples the risk of cancer so that women should be advised to get age-appropriate mammography. The medication is should not be used in patients with active hepatitis B infections. Vaccinations using living organisms are also contraindicated.

Seminars in Respiratory Disease

...

There are many other diseases of the nervous system that can affect the lungs. Most neurological disease cause a restrictive lung defect with a normal diffusion and subsequent hypercarbic respiratory failure. Others can cause dysfunction of swallowing and hence aspiration and pneumonia.

Poliomyelitis is a viral disease which, in one sense, was important in the development of respiratory therapy. The virus attacks the anterior horn of the spinal cord causing asymmetric, peripheral polyneuropathy which often involves the muscles of respiration resulting in respiratory failure. At one point in the 1950's, St. Mary's Hospital in Rochester, MN, then the largest hospital in the world, had an entire floor filled with patients on "iron lungs." The disease is to a large extent irreversible, and many children grew up in iron lungs. The Salk vaccine, developed in the early 1950's, changed the outlook for millions of children. But recently, the anti-vaccine campaign threatens to bring the world back into the Middle Ages. In addition, a new virus causing partially reversible polyneuropathy has appeared. Hopefully, we will soon have a vaccine to counteract that disease.

The use of non-invasive ventilation (NIV) both in hospital and at home is increasing rapidly. Not only can it be used in patients with neuromuscular disease, but recent studies have shown that it is effective in patients with respiratory failure from a host of conditions including COPD and congestive heart failure as well as in patients post-extubation. NIV reduces the work of breathing by applying positive end-expiratory pressure, increasing lung compliance, and reducing the threshold required to initiate a breath. It is contraindicated in patients with facial trauma or burns, fixed upper airway obstruction, vomiting, or after a cardiac arrest. Either a ventilator or a BiPAP device can be used. In the last five years NIV has been used to treat patients with COPD and an elevated $PaCO_2$ at home with significant improvement in one year mortality in several studies. It has been shown to increase survival in patients with ALS as well in several excellent studies.

Suggestions for minor papers

1. Compare Guillain-Barré, Myasthenia Gravis, ALS, and Multiple Sclerosis.
2. What parts of the nervous system do the neurological diseases we discussed involve?
3. What is the action potential? How is it transmitted down the nerve?
4. What are the functions of the myelin sheath?
5. How can NIV be used in the treatment of neuromuscular diseases?

Peter A. Petroff, MD

Nine

Cancer of the Lung

Cancers are diseases in which abnormal cells divide without regulation. Some cancer cells may appear normal under the microscope, but their genetic structure has changed enough so that they no longer respond to the tissue regulators which limit their growth and multiplication. Because of this they invade the surrounding normal tissue. In addition, the genetic change allows the cells to migrate by lymphatic channels or through the blood to other organs in the body.

Almost any cell can become a cancer cell. It is likely that we form cancer cells somewhere in our body every day. But our immune system is able to identify these cells as abnormal, attack them, and eliminate them. For a cancer cell to survive it must also have the ability to fool the immune system. In one sense, cancer is due to the failure of our immune system. Cancer cells actually fool the immune system into thinking that they are normal cells.

Cancer is the second most common cause of death in the United States. The most common cancers are cancers of the skin, but with the exception of melanomas, these cancers are rarely fatal. The most common fatal cancer in both men and women is lung cancer, most often caused by the use of tobacco. Lung cancer kills three times as many people as colon cancer, three times as many men as prostate cancer and four times as many women as breast cancer, the second commonest cause of cancer in women. Other common cancers include pancreatic cancer, prostate cancer, leukemias and lymphomas, liver cancer, ovarian cancer, and esophageal cancer.

While, in general, the treatment of cancer has improved dramatically over the last fifty years and people with cancer are living longer, most persons who get one of the common cancers listed above will die of their disease. In most of these cancers, such as colon cancer, breast cancer, prostate cancer, and even lung cancer, early detection is available which can save lives.

The treatment for most cancers is still surgery but chemotherapy and, most recently, immunotherapy has made impressive strides in the care of many of the fatal cancers.

Peter A. Petroff, MD

Case Presentations

1.

Tim K. comes to the pulmonary clinic because of a three-month history of cough. His cough is incessant, both night and day. It is productive of clear phlegm but on occasion Tim has noticed some "streaks of blood" mixed in the phlegm. His wife became concerned when he told her about the blood and arranged the visit to the clinic.

Tim will be sixty in a month. He has smoked since he was a teenager and smokes about a pack a day though he is trying to cut back. He has had a "smoker's cough" on most days for the last twenty years but tells the doctor, "This cough is different." The cough has become more frequent and more severe. "It wakes me at night." Tim also notes that he has lost about ten pounds in the last couple of months without trying. He has not had any chest pain, nor has he been short of breath, but his breathing was never exceptionally good. He can walk around easily at work but always takes the elevator to the second floor. "Walking up a flight of stairs makes me really short of breath. I have to stop and rest after walking up one flight."

He has no history of pneumonia or other lung disease. He has no history of heart disease. His past history is largely unremarkable. He drinks a martini every night. He takes medication for his blood pressure but has no drug allergies. He has never had surgery nor been in a hospital. He has worked as an accountant for all of his adult life. He hopes to retire next year. His parents both died of heart disease.

His physical examination shows him to be an alert, thin male in no respiratory distress. His pants are quite loose-fitting about the waist. His height is 5'10" and his weight 165 lbs. His BP is 124/60; his pulse is 82. His oxygen saturation is 94% on room air. Examination of his head and neck is unremarkable. The lungs are clear with markedly decreased breath sounds. At times, the doctor can hear a slight monophonic expiratory squeak over the right upper lobe posteriorly. The heart sounds are normal. The liver is normal in size. There is no pedal edema.

The doctor orders a chest radiograph and several laboratory studies.

The complete blood count shows mild erythrocytosis with a hemoglobin of 18.3 Gms. Normal hemoglobin is between 12-16. The chemistry profile and urinalysis are normal except for an elevated calcium of 11.5. Normal is less than 10.5. The chest radiograph shows a large right hilum with a mass-like lesion involving the proximal right upper lobe.

The patient returns after the tests and the doctor tells him he is concerned about the mass lesion. He suggests that Tim get a CAT scan with iodine contrast to get a better look at the lesion.

The CAT scan shows the right upper lobe mass. It measures about 2 cm in diameter. Surprisingly, there are no hilar nodes measuring more than 1 cm. in size. In addition, the subcarinal and paratracheal nodes are all normal in size. There are no other lesions in the lung, but the lung is emphysematous. The liver appears normal. The rest of the exam is normal.

After reviewing the CAT scan with Tim, the doctor says that he will need to find out what the mass is and whether it can be approached surgically. Tim needs to have pulmonary function testing as well as a bronchoscopy. Tim agrees to the procedures.

The pulmonary function testing shows:

FVC	3.5 liters	88% of predicted
FEV1	2.1 liters	70% of predicted
FEV1/FVC	60%	significantly decreased
MMF	1.5 liters/second	50% of predicted
TLC	6.0 liters	100% of predicted
RV	2.5 liters	125% of predicted
DCO	65% of predicted	

The bronchoscopy shows a friable grayish, glistening mass lesion about 1 and a half centimeters in size filling the anterior bronchus of the right upper lobe. The tracheal carina was sharp. The rest of the examination was normal. A biopsy of the lesion confirmed it was a squamous cell cancer of the lung.

Two days later Tim returned with his wife to discuss the findings. The doctor explains the findings which suggest the lesion could probably be removed surgically. The main concern was the pulmonary function. If the surgeon removed only the right upper lobe Tim would lose about a fifth of his lung function or about 0.7 liters of his FVC. He would have 2.8 liters left and an FEV1 of 1.7 liters. He would be shorter of breath but could function fairly well. He probably would not need oxygen. If on the other hand, the doctor had to take out the entire right lung, Tim would lose 1.8 liters of his vital capacity. He would then have a vital capacity of 1.7 liters and his FEV1 would only be 1 liter. He would likely be severely short of breath and probably would need oxygen after the surgery. Still the surgery could be done.

Tim asks about alternative therapies. The doctor explains that chemotherapy was rarely helpful in this type of cancer but sometimes radiation therapy could help him live a little longer. Neither therapy would cure the disease. The doctor leaves the room to allow Tim and his wife to discuss the findings. The doctor returns 15 minutes later, and Tim says he wants the surgery. The doctor orders laboratory testing for blood clotting as well as an EKG and schedules Tim for surgery the following week.

The surgeon performs a right upper lobectomy. The whole tumor is contained in just the right upper lobe and there is no evidence of lymphatic spread of the tumor. Tim was discharged three days later from the hospital. Follow-up six months later shows no evidence of tumor recurrence.

2.

Andres C. is a fifty-year-old male who comes to the internal medicine clinic because he is quite weak. He has been weak for several months. Now, he cannot even get up from a chair without help. He says, "My legs are like jelly. I even fell twice. I needed help to get up off the floor." He feels good otherwise. He says he is in good health "for a smoker." He has had a cough for several years, but he doesn't worry about it. He does not have any chest pain. He is not short of breath. He hasn't lost weight. His appetite is good.

He smokes about a pack and a half a day. He has smoked for more than thirty-five years. He does not drink. He takes the vitamins that his wife tells him to take. He has no allergies, surgery, or medical admissions. His family history is important. His father died with colon cancer at the age of 55. His mother is still living. The patient worked in a steel mill in South Bend, IN. from the time he was 17 until he was 25. He was an electrician. "I worked with the insulators." Afterwards, he went to college and since college he has worked as a laboratory technician.

His physical examination shows him to be a jovial, alert male in no distress. His face is plethoric, mildly Cushinoid in appearance. His legs are thin with a protuberant abdomen. He is 5'10" tall and weighs 210 lbs. His blood pressure is 178/108. His pulse is 86. His oxygen saturation is 96% on room air. Examination of his head and neck is normal. His lungs show symmetrically decreased breath sounds. The heart sounds are normal. The liver is enlarged; the liver edge is 8 cm below the right costal margin. The spleen tip is not palpable. There is slight edema in both feet.

The doctor orders a chest radiograph and laboratory.

The blood count is normal. The chemistry panel shows a sodium of 136 with a potassium of 2.8 (normal 3.5-4.4). The kidney tests are normal while the liver enzymes are twice normal. The chest radiograph shows a 4 cm right paratracheal mass lesion.

The patient returns after the laboratory tests. The doctor advises a CAT scan and additional laboratory to determine why the potassium is so low. The doctor says the weakness is due to the low potassium.

The CAT scan confirms the presence of the large right upper lobe mass lesion. In addition, there is a small nodule in the left lower lung field and several of the subcarinal nodes are larger than 1 cm. The CAT scan also showed several small mass lesions in the liver. The blood tests show a markedly elevated serum cortisol level.

After reviewing the tests, the doctor suggested a bronchoscopy to determine the type of lesion. He also begins Andres on high dose potassium.

The bronchoscopy shows a two-centimeter erythematous lesion along the right tracheal wall. Biopsies are done. There is a moderate amount of bleeding. The biopsies show *small cell cancer*.

Andres returns to see the doctor two days after the bronchoscopy. The doctor tells him he has an inoperable lung cancer but that small cell lung cancer often responds to chemotherapy. He also said that the low potassium was due to the tumor releasing a type of ACTH or adrenocortical trophic hormone which causes the adrenal gland to make cortisol. Cortisol causes the kidney to lose potassium. Andres asks about surgery. The doctor said it is just not possible.

Andres saw the oncologist and began taking chemotherapy. The tumor responded. Both the lung and liver lesions decreased in size over the next six months. The potassium improved but he told the doctor he "just wasn't as happy as I used to be."

Unfortunately, after two years of therapy the tumor became non-responsive to chemotherapy, and Andres was admitted to Hospice Care. He died after just a few weeks.

3.

Victoria C. is an extremely pleasant 65-year-old woman who is referred to the pulmonary clinic because she was found to have a small pulmonary nodule on a CAT scan of her abdomen which was done because of atypical abdominal pain. She had a cholecystectomy the year before which was uneventful. However, 4 months ago she began developing pain in her right upper quadrant of the abdomen. The pain was intermittent but occurred nearly every day; it was moderately severe and cramping in quality but was not associated with any other gastrointestinal or genitourinary symptoms such as nausea, diarrhea, hematuria, or urinary frequency. Her laboratory studies were normal as was an ultrasound of her liver and pancreas. Because of the persistence of the pain, a CAT scan of the abdomen was performed. The study was normal save for the presence of a 7 mm non-calcified nodule in the left lower lobe.

Victoria is a nurse who works at the clinic. She was born and raised in the Philippines but came to the United States at the age of twenty. She had a BCG vaccination as a child. She has had a positive PPD since then. She was exposed to active tuberculosis as a teenager. Her roommate in nursing school had tuberculosis. Victoria, however, was not ill at the time. She had a chest radiograph at the time which was normal. She also had a screening chest radiograph when she immigrated to the US. She has had annual chest radiographs at the clinic because of her positive PPD. All the chest x-rays were normal.

She has no unusual hobbies. She is not a spelunker. Nor does she raise pigeons or chickens. She lives in the suburbs with her husband. Her children are married but still live in the area. She travels home to visit her family in the Philippines about once a decade.

She has no pulmonary symptoms such as cough or dyspnea. She has not lost any weight. She has never smoked. Her husband smoked for about 2 years after they met but quit completely. Her past history is otherwise unremarkable. Her mother and father are both in their nineties and are healthy. She has five siblings none of whom have any pulmonary problems. Her brother died of colon cancer. The patient had a dysplastic (precancerous) colon polyp 5 years before, but subsequent colonoscopies have been negative.

She is alert but anxious. Her height is 5 feet, 4 inches. Her weight is 110 lbs. Her BP is 136/85. Her pulse is 86. Her O2 saturation is 98% on room air.

Her examination is totally normal. There are no skin nodules or abnormal discolorations. The lungs are clear with normal breath sounds. There is a soft grade 2/6 systolic murmur at the apex of the heart. She states she has had the murmur for years and a cardiac catheterization done ten years ago was normal. Her abdominal exam shows a normal sized liver and no abdominal masses. The abdominal pain is gone. There is no edema. Her peripheral pulses are normal.

After discussing the findings with the patient, the doctor sends her for a CAT scan of the chest with contrast as well as PFTs.

The CAT scan of the chest shows only the 7 mm nodule in the left lower lobe. The nodule cannot be seen on the screening chest radiograph done before the CAT scan. No other nodules are present. The nodule is not calcified and does not appear speculated. Pulmonary studies are normal.

The doctor orders a blood test for TB (Quantiferon Gold) because of the positive PPD. He also orders serology studies for coccidiomycosis and histoplasmosis. He tells her that, based on her age and the size of the nodule, her risk of cancer is about 3% or 1 in thirty. He suspects that, even though the nodule is not calcified, it is most likely a scar from tuberculosis.

The Quantiferon Gold test is normal as are the studies for fungi.

He states that the nodule is too small to be evaluated accurately with a PET scan and a biopsy will be very risky and likely not to be successful, again because of the small size of the nodule. He recommends a follow up CAT scan at 6 months to make sure the nodule is stable. She will have to have CAT scans again in one year and still another in two years. If all three studies are stable, surgery is very unlikely to be necessary and she can return to her annual chest radiographs as long as she continues to work at the clinic.

Victoria returns for each scheduled CAT scan. Over the two years, the nodule actually decreases slightly in size to 6 mm in diameter. The doctor tells her, "No further testing is needed."

Background for the presentations

The first patient has a squamous cell carcinoma of the lung associated with hypercalcemia. The hypercalcemia is likely paraneoplastic. This type of cancer can produce a form of PTH (parathyroid hormone) which stimulates the bones to release calcium. Surgery is the primary treatment for squamous cell carcinoma. The ectopic hormone production is <u>not</u> a sign of metastasis. The tumor is still operable even with hypercalcemia.

The second patient also has a type of paraneoplasia, this time due to a small cell lung cancer. Small cell cancers are the most common causes of "ectopic hormone production" and immune mediated paraneoplasia such as muscle weakness and neuropathies. Small cell carcinoma is always caused by smoking, is almost always fatal, and rarely can be treated surgically.

The third patient presents an interesting contrast. Isolated pulmonary nodules are becoming more and more frequent as smokers get screening CAT scans in order to detect lung cancer earlier. In fact, almost half of all patients who have a screening CAT scan have a pulmonary nodule. Generally, the nodules are benign (not cancerous) but need to be evaluated and followed. Common causes of an isolated pulmonary nodule should be looked for.

Important points

1. An elevated calcium level in a patient with cancer can be a sign of paraneoplasia.
2. Squamous cell lung cancer and small cell cancer are almost always due to smoking.
3. Squamous cell carcinomas of the lung are generally slow growing. They metastasize late and may cavitate. However, most are centrally located and are found late in their course making treatment difficult.
4. Small cell carcinomas can produce many different types of ectopic hormones including ACTH, FSH (follicular stimulating hormone) and ADH (antidiuretic hormone).
5. Small cell carcinoma grows rapidly and metastasizes early.
6. Treatment of a small cell carcinoma is almost always with chemotherapy and radiotherapy.
7. Screening for lung cancer among patients who smoke often shows a pulmonary nodule.
8. BCG vaccine decreases the risk of TBC significantly. It is used in countries where there is a high incidence of the disease such as the Philippines. It will cause the PPD to be positive for about 20 years. If the PPD is positive 40 years after the patient had a BCG, the BCG vaccine is probably NOT the cause of the positive PPD.
9. The Quantiferon Gold test is replacing the PPD as a screening test for TB in many clinics and hospitals. However, it has about a 20% false negative rate.

Discussion

Cancer is a malignant neoplasm. The word "neoplasm" means "a new growth." It can be benign like the skin tags we have on our body, or it can be malignant. A malignant lesion is a neoplasm with uncontrolled growth and the potential to spread to other sites in the body.

Lung cancers were rare before the year 1900. There were only 400 case reports up to that time. With the increasing popularity of cigarettes, the risk of lung cancer grew. By the early 1920's the relationship between smoking and lung cancer was well established but still, tobacco use skyrocketed.

Movie stars were paid to smoke on screen and in public. They became a role model for movie-goers who took up smoking to emulate their favorite star. Sales of tobacco soared. Even President Reagan advertised for "Lucky Strike" before he was president of course. I can remember him saying,

"LSMFT. Lucky Strike means fine tobacco." In 1964 the Surgeon General released its report linking tobacco and lung cancer. After the release of the report, sales of tobacco products began to fall off. Nevertheless, smoking is still acceptable in many parts of the world and lung cancer is still a major problem. In 2017, there were about 225,000 new cases and 150,000 deaths from lung cancer in the United States. However, more and more individuals who get cancer are ex-smokers or never smokers. The lifetime risk of getting lung cancer is about 8% in men and 6% in women. Worldwide the numbers are staggering. Tobacco smoking continues to increase in the Middle East and Africa. Two-thirds of Chinese doctors are smokers! But there is some good news even in China. Smoking in China has decreased 30% over the last thirty years. In 2012 there were 1,800,000 new cases of lung cancer and 1,590,000 deaths from the disease world-wide. About 17% of Americans and 27% of Europeans smoke. One statistic that emphasizes the enormity of the problem: more people died of lung cancer in the United States in the last 5 years than in all the wars in our history!

The main risk factor for developing lung cancer is smoking. Even second-hand and third-hand smoke cause cancer. Second-hand smoke occurs when a non-smoker is exposed on a regular basis to smoking at home, in the car, or at work by an active smoker. Third-hand smoke is the smoking residue left on clothes, furniture, curtains, and other household items by tobacco smoke. Smokers (including ex-smokers) are ten times (the risk ratio is 10) more likely to get lung cancer than never smokers. Second-hand smoke increases the risk of cancer by 30% (the risk ratio is 1.3). Tobacco smoke causes chromosome mutations, about 1 mutation for every 15 cigarettes smoked. There are more than 60 carcinogens in cigarette smoke. Filters were meant to decrease the cancer risk, but the first filters were made with asbestos fiber which is, of course, a carcinogen. More than 85% of lung cancers are due to smoking.

Other risk factors include exposure to asbestos, arsenic in workers making pesticides and paints, chromium, mustard gas, and polycyclic aromatic hydrocarbons in foundry workers. Ionizing radiation also poses a significant risk. Even CAT scans significantly increase the risk of cancer. Radon gas, naturally occurring in the soil, may account for about 2% of lung cancers. In addition, certain families appear predisposed to developing lung cancer. A first degree relative of a person with lung cancer has twice to thrice the risk of developing cancer. Several foci have been identified on chromosomes as possible culprits, but no definite genetic pattern has been established.

Asbestos is the most studied occupational cause of lung cancer. By itself, it causes a five-fold increase in the risk of cancer but when an asbestos worker smokes the risk of cancer is increased fifty-fold! Asbestos also causes mesotheliomas, which are tumors of the pleural lining of the lung and peritoneal lining in the abdomen. The asbestos fiber causes all the common types of lung cancer.

All lung cancer cells have an abnormal genetic structure. These changes result in the production of growth factors which encourage the rapid multiplication of the tumor cells. At the same time, the genes responsible for limiting growth (tumor-suppression genes or "checkpoints") are turned off. As the tumor grows it sends signals to the surrounding tissue to make more blood vessels which will help it meet its metabolic needs (angiogenesis). The genes must also turn off the cellular mechanism for the aging and death (called *apoptosis*) of the cancer cells. Finally, the genes must allow the tumor to spread or metastasize and release additional chemicals which impair the immune system.

Some investigators speculate that each cancer has a primordial cell or "stem cell." It is the stem cell that is responsible for the genetic changes which causes the tumor to grow, invade healthy tissue and metastasize.

There are two major types of lung cancer based on immunohistochemistry staining as well as the presence of certain molecular markers. Small cell lung cancers (SCLC) consist of masses of tiny cells with scant cytoplasm with small darkly stained nuclear inclusions. These cells are characterized by the presence of neuro-endocrine molecular markers. Under the microscope they look like a bowl of Quaker Oats. These cells were thought at one time to be derived from the K cells or Kulchinsky cells, remnants of primitive neuroendocrine cells, found along the basement membrane. Small cell cancers make up about 14% of all lung cancers. Typically, these cancers present as a central mass lesion. They grow rapidly, doubling in size every two months and spread early. By the time of initial presentation more than 90% of small cell lung cancers have already spread to other organs.

The adenocarcinomas, squamous cell carcinomas and the large cell carcinomas are lumped together to form the non-small cell cancers (NSCLC). The most common lung cancer at the present time by far is the adenocarcinoma. This is a major change since the 1960's. Adenocarcinomas most often have a gland-like appearance under the microscope with evidence of mucin production. Most adenocarcinomas are derived from the mucous glands that line the smaller airways. They have become the most common form of lung cancer, accounting for almost half of all lung cancers. These cancers often present as discrete peripheral nodules. However, they metastasize rapidly. Nevertheless, because they are peripheral in location, they offer the best hope at long time cure. However, one subclass of adenocarcinomas is quite different. It used to be called the bronchioloalveolar carcinoma but is now classified as the *lepidic* subgroup of adenocarcinoma. These cancers develop from the alveolar type 2 cells and appear microscopically as sheets of alveolar type 2 cells lining the inside of alveoli. Often these patient present with a cough productive a copious amount of clear, surfactant filled mucous. These tumors can present as diffuse multifocal disease or as a slow growing solitary nodule.

Squamous cell carcinomas appear as sheets of abnormal squamous cells, the same type of cells that make up our skin. These cells are derived from metaplastic ("changed tissue") of the trachea and large bronchi. Smoking causes the pseudostratified columnar epithelium to disappear and be replaced by squamous cells (metaplasia). Over time, they become abnormal or dysplastic and finally cancerous. Squamous cell cancers account for 20-25% of all lung cancers. These cancers are generally centrally located, slow growing tumors that metastasize late. They may cavitate. Because they are generally central in location, they are often large tumors when they first present and are generally inoperable.

Large cell cancers consist of masses of primitive large cells that have none of the features of the other types of cancer cells. These tumors may be derived from the lung's own primitive stem cell. They account for only a small percentage, about 3%, of lung cancers. These tumors are fast-growing and spread rapidly. They occur in heavy smokers. They have a two to one male predominance and are invariably fatal.

Lung cancers can present in several ways. If the lesion is centrally located in the trachea or a major airway, it can present with **local symptoms** such as cough or hemoptysis or symptoms of bronchial obstruction such as a pneumonia or atelectasis. If the tumor is in the parenchyma of the lung, it will grow until it invades the pleura or pericardium, invades the phrenic nerve, blocks the superior vena cava, or damages the recurrent laryngeal nerve. The tumor can also present with **metastatic disease** involving the brain, liver, bones, or lung. Lastly it can present with **paraneoplastic syndrome**. More than half of the patients have advanced disease when they become symptomatic.

The most common local symptom presentation is a new cough or a change in a cough. Hemoptysis, chest pain, wheezing, and stridor are much less frequently seen. If the tumor invades the pleural space, pleurisy or shortness of breath may occur. If the tumor involves the pericardium, the patient may present with cardiac arrhythmias, especially atrial arrhythmias such as atrial fibrillation. Involvement of the pericardium may also cause pericardial tamponade due to the pericardial space being filled with blood. If the tumor involves the phrenic nerve ipsilateral diaphragmatic paralysis with shortness of breath will result. If the tumor involves the left main stem bronchus it may damage the recurrent laryngeal nerve and cause hoarseness. If the tumor is located along the right side of the trachea, it can compress the superior vena cava causing swelling and duskiness of the face and right arm. Tumors that form in the apex of a lung, called Pancoast tumors, often involve the brachial plexus causing shoulder and arm pain. They can also involve the sympathetic fibers which supply the ipsilateral face and cause drooping eyelid (ptosis), a small pupil (miosis), and absent sweating (anhidrosis) on one side of the face.

Extrathoracic metastatic disease is quite common. Fifty percent of patients with squamous cell cancer, 80% with adenocarcinoma, and 95% of patients with a small call cancer have metastatic disease at autopsy. Many patients present with metastatic disease as their first symptom. The patient may present with a stroke due to a brain lesion, jaundice, and liver failure due to liver metastasis, or bone pain or a fracture due to metastatic bone lesions.

Paraneoplastic symptoms are much less common. By themselves they do not mean that the tumor is inoperable. The most serious paraneoplastic syndrome is hypercalcemia due to ectopic parathyroid hormone secretion. This is most often seen with squamous cell cancer. The hypercalcemia causes weakness, constipation, nausea, and confusion. Most of the other paraneoplastic syndromes are seen with small cell cancers. These include ectopic secretion of antidiuretic hormone which causes severe hyponatremia (low sodium), ectopic adrenocorticotrophic hormone which causes increased levels of cortisol and hypokalemia. Some tumors also secrete follicular stimulating hormone which causes gynecomastia. Large cell lung tumors secrete a subunit of human chorionic gonadotropin which leads to high levels of estrogens and painful gynecomastia.

Other paraneoplastic symptoms and findings include clubbing of the fingers which is found in the non-small cell group of cancers, especially squamous cell cancer, generalized weakness, fatigue, fever, and abnormal clotting. The patient may be hypercoagulable and present with thrombophlebitis or a pulmonary embolism. One very interesting symptom is the Eaton-Lambert syndrome which is associated with small cell lung cancer. It is a neuromuscular junction disorder which affects the communication between nerves and muscles, driven by the development of antibodies that target calcium channels on the presynaptic nerve terminals. This decreases the releases of the acetylcholine neurotransmitter is reduced. The main symptoms are muscle weakness and areflexia but unlike myasthenic gravis, with repeated use, the muscle gets stronger. Just as with myasthenia, Eyelid drooping, Fatigue, Trouble speaking and swallowing may occur as may erectile dysfunction and tingling in the extremities and bladder and bowel changes.

Workup of the suspected lung cancer patient involves chest radiography, a CAT scan of the chest as well as laboratory studies to look for anemia, thrombocytopenia, hypercalcemia, and changes in the sodium and potassium levels. The CAT scan of the lung is the most important step in determining the stage of the cancer and answering the question, "Can this patient have surgery?" Pulmonary function testing also should be done as well as a cardiac evaluation including an EKG.

Obtaining tissue is the key to the diagnoses of lung cancer. The tissue can be obtained through a bronchoscope if the lesion is centrally located or by a percutaneous needle biopsy if the lesion is in the parenchyma of the lung and out of reach of the bronchoscope. A core or large biopsy is best in order to do molecular staging. In addition, gene testing of the tumor is done to determine the best type of chemotherapy as well as the likelihood the tumor will respond to chemotherapy.

Once the diagnosis is made the patient must be staged. If the lesion is a small cell carcinoma there are only two stages: limited disease and extensive disease. Limited disease is a disease confined to an area of the chest that can be encompassed by a single focal area of radiation. Generally, this means the lesion is unilateral without evidence of spread outside the hemothorax. But disease can also be located around the trachea and involve the recurrent laryngeal nerve in the left hemithorax and the superior vena cava in the right hemithorax and still be able to be treated with focal radiation. This is still considered limited disease. Anything more than this is extensive. Many oncologists recommend getting a PET scan to identify any metastasis as well as a CAT scan of the brain in all patients with small cell cancer.

Staging the non-small cell carcinomas involves looking at the size of the tumor (T), whether the tumor involves the lymph nodes (N), and whether the tumor has metastasized (M). For example, T1 tumors are less than 3 cm in diameter, T 2 tumors are 3-5 cm in diameter, T3 tumors are 5-7 cm in diameter, and T4 tumors are more than 7 cm in diameter. N0 tumors have no lymph node involvement while N1 involve the hilar lymph nodes on the same side of the lesion. N2 tumors show lymph nodes in the mediastinum, again on the ipsilateral side while N3 tumors have contralateral lymph nodes. M0 means no evidence of metastasis while M1 means distant metastasis. Based on the TNM classification, the tumors are then staged. Stage 1 cancer is cancer that has not spread to any lymph node. Stage 2 cancer has spread to adjacent intrapulmonary or hilar lymph nodes. Stage 3a cancer has spread to lymph nodes, but all the lymph nodes are in the ipsilateral hemithorax. All three of these stages are operable. Stage 3b involves lymph nodes on the contralateral hemithorax and stage 4 is cancer with distant metastasis. Stage 3b and 4 are inoperable.

Treatment of small cell cancer is largely with chemotherapy. If a tiny lesion is found without any evidence of metastases, surgery may be an option. That is very, very unusual.

Treatment of non-small cell cancer is almost always surgery if surgery is possible. If the patient's disease is extensive, if there is a pleural effusion with cancer cells found in the fluid, if the tumor involves the recurrent laryngeal nerve, the superior vena cava, the heart or mediastinum, surgery is impossible. Similarly, if the predicted post-operative FEV1 is less than a liter or if the patient has had a heart attack in the last three months surgery is contraindicated or will leave the patient totally incapacitated. When these contraindications to surgery are present the patient can be treated with radiation and, in some cases, chemotherapy. In addition, more and more therapy is directed at molecular targeting—attacking the chemicals within cells that drive growth (tyrosine kinase) and prevent the immune system from destroying the cancer. Bevacizumab is an antibody that inhibits vascular endothelial growth factor while pembrolizumab is an antibody, a checkpoint inhibitor, which turns on the immune response directed against the cancer.

The life expectancy of a patient with limited small cell cancer is about two years while with extensive small cell cancer it is about a year. A few percent of patient with limited disease are alive at 5 years. The survival rate for patients with operable non-small cell cancer is about 50%. The overall 5-year survival rate with lung cancer is about 18.6% which is much lower than breast cancer at 90%, colon cancer at 64% and prostate cancer at 98%. The survival rate for lung cancer was 11% fifty years ago. It has hardly improved. More than half of patients with lung cancer die in their first year after diagnosis.

Because of the terrible outlook for patients with lung cancer, the use of screening to detect early cancer has been a long-term goal of pulmonologists and epidemiologists. In the 1960's and 1970's the use of chest radiographs combined with sputum cytology was tried in seven large studies. None showed any mortality benefit. More recently, screening has been done with low dose chest helical non-contrast CAT scans. Several trials, both in Europe and the United States, have shown that early lung cancer can be detected by this method and mortality can be reduced. People who smoke or who quit smoking within the past 15 years, have a 30 pack-year smoking history and are over 55 years of age and under 75 were studied. The study showed that 320 patients had to be screened to prevent one cancer death. However, there were a large number of false positives. In fact, when a nodule 4 mm in diameter was considered positive, there was a 94% false positive rate. False positives are patients with nodules that are not due to cancer. Moreover, the rate of detection did not decrease over time meaning that the patients who had a nodule on the first exam would have to get a CAT scan every year for the rest of their lives.

Suggestions for minor papers

1. Why is pulmonary function testing important in the treatment of lung cancer?
2. What does paraneoplasia mean? What are some examples?
3. Discuss staging of lung tumors.
4. Compare the four common types of lung cancer.
5. Discuss how immune therapy is changing the treatment for lung cancer.
6. Compare first-hand, second-hand, and third-hand smoking.
7. Discuss the use of the BCG vaccine in developing countries. Should it be used in the developed world such as the USA and Europe? If not, why not?
8. What are the indications for treatment of the patient with a positive PPD?

Peter A. Petroff, MD

Ten

Diseases of the Pleura

The pleural space is a virtual space between two thin layers of mesothelial cells, one of which lines the inside of the thoracic cage and is called the parietal pleura and the other of which completely covers the lungs with the exception of the hila and is called the visceral pleura. Underlying the mesothelial cells is a thin layer of fibrous tissue which contain lymphatics, blood vessels, and **only below the parietal pleura**, sensory nerves. In addition, the parietal pleura has holes between some of the mesothelial cells, called "stomata," which allow fluid to pass from the pleural space directly into the underlying lymphatics.

The parietal pleura's vascular system is part of the systemic circulation. The arteries arise from the intercostal arteries and the veins drain into the systemic venous system. On the other hand, the visceral pleura's vascular system is more complex. Its arteries also get blood from the systemic circulation, but the blood is from the bronchial arteries which arise from the aorta. Its veins drain into the pulmonary venous system.

Normally, the pleural space contains only a few ccs of fluid, about 20 ccs in all. But fluid constantly pours into the pleural space and must be resorbed into the lymphatics of the parietal pleura. The lymph channels ultimately drain into the thoracic duct and are returned to the circulation. Normally, fluid resorption is equal to fluid formation. Thus, there is no accumulation of fluid in the space.

But for 1,600,000 Americans fluid does accumulate in the pleural space. Sometimes the amount of fluid is massive, more than three or four liters, completely or nearly completely, filling the thoracic cavity resulting in chest discomfort and shortness of breath. Sometimes the fluid accumulation is small, found incidentally on a chest radiograph. The cause of the pleural effusion or hydrothorax must always be found.

On the other hand, about 40,000 Americans a year, develop air in the pleural space, a condition called a pneumothorax. Half the time it is due to medical misadventure; half the time it is due to either injury or illness. Either way the cause must be found and the pneumothorax treated.

Peter A. Petroff, MD

Case Presentations

1.

Julius M., a sixty-four-year-old male, comes to the emergency room because of shortness of breath and vague chest discomfort. He states he was totally well until two months ago when he began to notice he was breathless going for his morning walk. The shortness of breath gradually became worse and worse. After about six weeks he decided to quit smoking to see if that might help. He smoked about a pack a day for the last fifty years. But quitting smoking didn't help a bit. In fact, he began to notice fullness in the right side of his chest. He had a hard time describing the discomfort. It really was not "pain." It did not hurt to turn or to breath. The right side of his chest just felt heavy.

Julius said he had pneumonia many years before and had to be hospitalized. He had a cough with thick yellow phlegm. "A smoker's cough, doc." He never coughed up blood nor did he have fever, chills, or night sweats. He grew up on a farm, but his family moved to the city when he was quite young. He worked off and on in construction. Sometimes he worked as a roofer; sometimes he worked as a carpenter. He was never a painter or insulator. He did mostly residential construction. He never worked at industrial sites.

He drank about three beers a day. He didn't take any medicines and had no drug allergies. He had a cholecystectomy three or four years ago. His father and mother both died of congestive heart failure.

His examination showed him to be alert and in no distress. He was fairly muscular. He was not dyspneic at rest. His weight was 248 lbs. His height was 6'2." His blood pressure was 155/85 and his pulse was 76. He was afebrile.

Examination of his head and neck was unremarkable. Examination of his chest revealed that the right hemithorax did, in fact, appear larger than the left. It did not expand and contract with inspiration and exhalation. The percussion note was flat over the entire right hemithorax. There were no breath sounds on the right at all. The breath sounds on the left were diminished with prolonged expiration.

The liver edge was 6 cm below the right costal margin, but the liver was not enlarged to percussion. The abdominal exam was otherwise unremarkable. There was no edema in the lower extremities. There were no pedal pulses.

The emergency physician asked for a chest x-ray.

The chest x-ray showed that the entire right hemithorax was filled with fluid and the heart and trachea were shifted to the left.

The ER doctor told Julius he needed to be admitted to hospital. He then ordered several laboratory tests including a complete blood count, chemistry profile, C-reactive protein, urinalysis, coagulation studies including a PT and PTT as well as an EKG. *All the tests were normal.* While Julius was waiting for a hospital bed, the ER doctor performed a thoracentesis. He obtained more than three liters of fluid from Julius' chest. The fluid was sent for several studies including a complete blood count and differential, glucose, LDH, protein, cytology, gram stain and culture, and an AFB smear and culture for tuberculosis.

After the procedure Julius told the doctor, "The weird feeling in my chest is gone! Thanks doc."

The doctor sent Julius to radiology for a CAT scan of the chest. From there, Julius went directly to his room in the ICU.

Later that day, the hospitalist, who would care for Julius while he was in the hospital, visited. He had some very bad news. The CAT scan showed that the fluid was gone, "All except a very tiny amount." But the radiologist saw a large lump in the middle of the right lower lobe. "It didn't look good." The doctor recommended a biopsy. Julius quickly agreed to the procedure which was done later that day.

The next morning the hospitalist returned with all the lab results. *The pleural fluid glucose was low at 43, the protein was quite high at 3.8 grams (normal is less than 3.0), the LDH was 150 (the serum LDH was 180), the smears were negative for bacteria and TB, but the cytology showed cancer cells, consistent with a squamous cell carcinoma as was the biopsy of the nodule in the chest.*

The doctor said that because the pleural fluid had cancer cells, chemotherapy was the best treatment and, if Julius agreed, he would call a cancer specialist to see him. Julius reluctantly agreed.

The next day, Julius told his doctor that the feeling in his chest had returned. The doctor ordered another chest radiograph which showed about a liter of fluid in the right chest. After discussing the situation with Julius and the oncologist, the doctor asked a surgeon to place a catheter through Julius' chest wall with one end in the pleural space and the other end in the peritoneal space which would allow the fluid to drain from the thorax into the abdomen.

The oncologist began Julius on chemotherapy which Julius tolerated well. He was discharged home. A home health nurse would visit him at least three times a week.

2.

Erin was a 72-year-old biker who was brought to the emergency room after she and the Harley Davidson she was piloting were struck nearly head on, by a drunk, driving in the wrong lane. The drunk was not injured and fled the scene but was later arrested.

On arrival in the ER, Erin was clearly in pain. Despite restraints she was agitated and barely responsive. The emergency technicians had placed a neck brace to prevent head movement. No sedation had been given. She was receiving 100% oxygen via a face mask. Her blood pressure was barely palpable at 80 systolic. Her pulse rate was 146. Her SaO2 was 86%.

The triage physician inserted a large bore IV into her right forearm and quickly examined her. Erin was dyspneic, struggling to breathe. She had a laceration with bruising on the left side of her head. Her hair was matted in blood. There was marked bruising over the right chest wall and the doctor could feel subcutaneous crepitus just below the clavicle. There was also tenderness over the upper rib cage. Breath sounds were absent over the entire right lung. The doctor placed his finger in the suprasternal notch. The trachea was shifted to the left. Examination of the abdomen showed moderate generalized tenderness with abdominal distension. The right foot was angled outward suggesting a hip fracture.

The physician called for a "stat" chest radiograph, but Erin's condition deteriorated rapidly. Her blood pressure cratered. He immediately inserted a large bore chest tube into the right chest wall in the 4th interspace near the midline. As he cut through the skin into the pleural space, there was a loud puff of air, as if a balloon suddenly deflated. Quickly he inserted the chest tube and connected it to an underwater seal. Erin's breathing instantly improved; her blood pressure rose to over a hundred; the trachea returned to a normal midline location.

The chest radiograph showed the chest tube in good position. The pneumothorax was gone. There were six pairs of rib fractures, from ribs two to seven on the right. There was also subcutaneous air along the right lateral and anterior chest wall extending into the neck as well as mediastinal air.

The triage physician continued the IV fluids at 200 ccs/hour and the oxygen at 2 l/min per nasal cannula. Her O2 saturation was 94%. He ordered a stat CBC, chemistry profile, PT, PTT, ABGs, cross table x-ray of Erin's neck, a CAT scan of her head and abdomen and an x-ray of her right hip.

Within an hour, Erin returned to the ER. *Her hemoglobin was 8 gms/100 cc. The rest of the CBC and chemistry profile was normal. The CAT scan of the brain was normal. There was no subdural hematoma. The x-ray of her neck was normal. There were no fractured cervical vertebrae. The abdominal CAT scan, however, showed a ruptured liver, likely due to one of the rib fractures and the x-ray of the right hip showed a fracture of the upper femur, just below the neck of the femur.* A surgical consultant was asked to see the patient.

Erin was taken to the surgical suite. The surgeon sutured the tear in the liver and placed a mesh over the area. He inserted a drain below the liver to prevent fluid buildup. She was admitted to the surgical intensive care unit where she was seen by the intensivist who would care for her while she was in the SICU. Over the next two hours she gradually awakened. She was given appropriate pain medicine and sedation to keep her comfortable. Intermittent compressive stockings were begun to prevent a blood clot.

The chest tube continued to leak. Moreover, despite a 40% Ventimask, the SaO2 remained in the 88-90% range. There was a definite paradoxical rib movement on the right consistent with a flail chest. After discussion with the patient, she was begun on non-invasive positive pressure assist. Her peak pressure was set at 25 cm with a PEEP of 10 cm. Almost at once, the flailing was diminished and the SaO2 improved to 95% though the air leak became a little worse.

The next day (Day 2 of admission), the orthopedic surgeon operated on the fractured hip under Propofol anesthesia. The patient was awake within a few minutes after the surgery and returned to the ICU. Pain medicines and sedation were continued.

The patient improved steadily. The pleural leak persisted but oxygenation remained excellent. There was no further abdominal bleeding, and the abdominal drain was removed on the next day.

By the fourth day, the leak had begun to diminish. When the non-invasive ventilation (NIV) was paused, however, it was clear the flail was still a problem. Supportive care continued over the next two days. Finally, on the seventh day the flailing stopped, and the NIV was discontinued. The air leak became minimal. The following day (Day 8) the leak stopped completely. The chest x-ray showed the lung fully expanded. The chest wall suction was discontinued, but the underwater seal was left overnight. The chest x-ray was repeated the following morning. The lung remained fully expanded. The chest tube was removed.

The patient continued to improve and was transferred to rehabilitation the following morning.

3.

Harvey C. is a very pleasant 78-year-old man who visits his primary doctor because of left shoulder pain. He tells the doctor, "I think it's arthritis, but it's not like my usual kind of arthritis." He says the pain is at the top of the shoulder and travels down his arm into his left hand. The pain is constant and is a burning pain. Raising, lowering, or rotating his left arm does not affect the pain. When the doctor has the patient raise and lower his arms, the range of motion is the same in both shoulders. Harvey also says he has lost some weight as well over the last few months. In fact, he has lost 15 lbs. without trying to lose weight. He also states, "I just don't feel good, doc."

The patient smoked about a pack a day for 40 years. He quit when he was sixty-five. He has no cough or phlegm. He is short of breath with moderate exertion, such as walking up one flight of stairs. He is shorter of breath than his wife. He has no history of pneumonia or other lung disease. He has no history of heart disease.

His past history is otherwise unremarkable. He drinks one beer a week. He takes Vasotec and hydrochlorothiazide for his blood pressure. He has not had any surgery and has never been in the hospital, in fact. His parents are dead. Both died with heart disease in their eighties. His brother and sister are alive and well.

The doctor then takes a social history. The patient lives with his wife in a nearby town. He has lived there all his life. He worked in a pharmacy as a teenager, then became an electrician. He did mainly industrial work in power plants, chemical plants, and a few refineries. He worked for forty years from the time he was 20 until he retired at 60. Now, he plays golf about once a week and fishes most days at a nearby lake.

The examination reveals Harvey to be alert, mildly obese in no acute respiratory distress. The doctor notices that Harvey is short of breath just taking off his clothes. The blood pressure is 126/84, the pulse is 88 and the oxygen saturation is 92% at rest.

Examination of the head and neck reveals a palpable hard mass in the left supraclavicular space. Examination of the lungs shows symmetrically decreased breath sounds with fine inspiratory crackles at both lung bases. The examination of the heart, abdomen and extremities is normal.

The doctor asks Harvey to get several blood tests and a chest radiograph (PAL).

The blood tests including the complete blood count and chemistry profile are normal, except for a mild anemia which appears to be a "normochromic" anemia (The red cells appear normal in size). The chest radiograph shows a large mass involving the left upper lobe and extending into the supraclavicular space. The mass on the chest radiograph correlates with the mass the doctor felt on examination. The mass appears to involve several of the ribs which appear to be "moth eaten." There are also bibasilar interstitial changes consistent with pulmonary fibrosis and several small calcified pleural plaques.

The doctor reviews the findings with Harvey. He recommends that Harvey have a biopsy of the mass in the supraclavicular space. Harvey agrees.

The biopsy of the mass, done by the radiologist using ultrasound guidance, is a mesothelioma which is a cancer involving the pleural lining. The doctor recommends that Harvey get a thorough cardiac evaluation and pulmonary function testing.

The cardiologist performs a chemical stress test which is normal. The pulmonary function testing reveals that the TLC, RV, FRC, VC and FEV1 are all reduced about 20% below predicted. The FEV1 is 2.1 liters. The predicted normal for an 80-year-old man who is 68 inches tall is 2.54 liters. The patient's six-minute walk is normal.

The doctor discusses the treatment of mesotheliomas with Harvey, "There are three options. The first is simply pain medication. The second is radiation and chemotherapy. The third is radiation followed by radical surgery. Life expectancy with pain medication alone is only a year or two. Radiation and chemotherapy will shrink the tumor and Harvey might live a few years more but the chances of living longer than 5 years is less than 10%. Surgical treatment is high risk and must be done in a specialized center. That surgery can be curative and may be worth the risk."

Harvey says he will discuss the treatment with his wife and family before deciding. A week later Harvey calls the doctor and says he wants to see the surgeon. The doctor arranges the appointment.

The surgeon sends Harvey for a CAT scan as well as a PET scan which shows the tumor, while large, is operable but he will have to remove two of Harvey's ribs along with the tumor. The tumor also involves the nerves to the hand and the doctor may have to remove the nerves. The nerves are sensory nerves and, while Harvey will have numbness in parts of his arm, he will be able to use his hand normally,.

The surgery is done two weeks later. Harvey's recovery is uneventful. One year after surgery there is no evidence of tumor recurrence.

Background for the presentations

The three cases represent three different types of pleural disease. The first is a case of a large pleural effusion due to lung cancer involving the pleura. The second represents a pneumothorax due to multiple rib fractures, which was complicated by a flail chest. The third case is of a tumor derived from the mesothelial cells of the pleura.

One of the important questions in the first case is whether the patient should have been given a sclerosing agent like talc rather than have a tunneling procedure. The question in the second case is simply how long can a leak persist before surgery is done to close it? The third case is that of a malignant tumor of the pleura, called a mesothelioma. Ninety-nine percent of these tumors are due to exposure to asbestos. The treatment of these tumors is radical surgery though most patients are too old or impaired to survive the surgery.

Important points

1. There are two large categories of pleural effusions: transudative and exudative.
2. The most common cause of a transudative pleural effusion is congestive heart failure.
3. The most common cause of an exudative pleural effusion is pneumonia.
4. A patient who has lung cancer and a pleural effusion may still be operable if there are no cancer cells in the pleural fluid.
5. Flail chest occurs when there are at least three contiguous ribs broken in at least two places. A "sternal flail' has three contiguous ribs broken on both sides of the sternum.
6. NIV (non-invasive ventilation) is an excellent treatment for flail chest and frequently reduces the need for intubation.
7. Hypoxemia in a patient with a flail chest injury is usually due to an underlying lung contusion.
8. Mesotheliomas are malignant tumors of the pleura.
9. Almost all mesotheliomas are due to exposure to the asbestos fiber which can even be quite minimal.

Discussion

The pleural space is a virtual space that lies between two layers of mesothelial cells and their supporting fibrous tissue. Normally, the space contains no more than 20 cc of fluid which acts as a lubricant for the lungs to expand and contract inside the more rigid chest wall. Surprisingly, not all animals have virtual pleural spaces. Elephants don't. And human beings who have had a pleurodesis, a procedure in which the virtual space is eliminated, do quite well without it.

While there are only a few ccs of fluid in the pleural space that does not mean that the space is static. It is, in fact, a dynamic space with fluid flowing into and out of the space continually.

Just like the relationship between capillaries and their surround interstitial space, the Starling equation also applies to the fluid shifts in the pleural space:

$$F = K \{(Ph\ c - Ph\ ip) - s\ (Posm\ c - Posm\ ip)\}$$

F is the fluid movement, K is the "filtration coefficient" (permeability), Ph is the hydrostatic pressure, s is the capillary permeability to protein, and Posm is the osmotic pressure. The little "c" refers to the capillary and the "ip" to pleural space.

When the chest cavity is opened, the chest wall expands and the lung collapses. Thus, in the closed chest, there is a negative pressure of about 5 cm holding the lung and chest wall together. Thus, we can calculate the fluid movement:

At the parietal pleura:

Ph c	=	30 cm H2O
Ph is	=	-5 cm
Posm c	=	32 cm
Posm is	=	6 cm

The driving pressure for the flux or fluid movement is (30 - -5) – 1 (32-6) or 9 cm H2O on the parietal pleura side of the virtual space. The main driving force accounting for this is the large hydrostatic pressure. The hydrostatic pressure is much lower on the visceral pleural side of the virtual space and the fluid movement is minimal. The flux is nearly zero. Most of the fluid in the pleural space normally comes from the parietal pleura.[5]

The fluid is absorbed by the stomata found in the parietal pleura which drain directly into the lymphatics and then to the thoracic duct.

Pleural fluid accumulation, called a pleural effusion, can result from either change in the visceral or parietal pleural capillary or osmotic pressure, or a change in the permeability constant. A change in the capillary pressure results in a *transudate*, fluid which is low in protein, while a change in the permeability results in an *exudate*, which is high in protein.

But these are just two of the possible mechanisms that can cause pleural fluid to accumulate. A third mechanism is due to the presence of tiny intradiaphragmatic channels communicating between the peritoneal cavity and the thoracic cavity. Since the pleural space has a more negative pressure than

---

[5] Weinberger, Cockrill, and Mandell: Principles of Pulmonary Medicine 7th edition, Elsevier, Philadelphia, 2019, pages 207-208.

the peritoneal cavity, ascites or peritoneal fluid (fluid in the abdominal cavity) will be drawn into the chest cavity because of the pressure gradient. This is most often seen in patients with cirrhosis of the liver. But inflammatory abdominal lesions such as pancreatitis can also cause this to happen.

In addition, parietal lymphatics can be obstructed by cancer cells or inflammation, which then prevents the resorption of the pleural fluid. Finally, the presence of inflammatory cells such as neutrophils, as in an empyema, or lymphocytes, as in tuberculosis or rheumatoid arthritis, or the presence of cancer cells in the pleural space will all cause an exudative pleural effusion.

Some Causes of Pleural Effusions[6]

Transudative effusions
    Congestive heart failure
    Cirrhosis
    Nephrotic syndrome
    Peritoneal dialysis
    Hypoalbuminemia (typical serum albumin, <1.5 mg/dl)
    Atelectasis
    Superior vena cava obstruction
    Trapped lung
    Sarcoidosis
    Myxedema
    Cerebrospinal fluid leak or ventriculopleural shunt
    Pulmonary arterial hypertension
    Pulmonary embolism
    Pericardial disease

Exudative effusions
    Infectious: bacterial, viral, tuberculosis-related, fungal, parasitic
    Neoplastic: metastatic disease (e.g., lung cancer, breast cancer, lymphoma
    Paramalignant effusions
    Reactive: reactive pleuritis due to underlying pneumonia (i.e., parapneumonic)
    Pulmonary embolism
    Pancreatitis, cholecystitis, hepatic or splenic abscess,
    Autoimmune disease such as rheumatoid arthritis and systemic lupus erythematosus,
    Medications including nitrofurantoin, methysergide, amiodarone, methotrexate, Dilantin
    Hemothorax
    Chylothorax
    Sarcoidosis
    Cholesterol effusions
    Asbestos pleural effusion

The most common cause of a transudate is congestive heart failure. Likely, the lungs become swollen with edematous fluid and behave like a wet sponge oozing fluid when they are squeezed.

The most common cause of an exudative pleural effusion is pneumonia. Pneumonia can cause a pleural effusion in two separate ways. It can cause a sterile inflammatory reaction which is called a

---

[6] Feller-Kopman, Light, Ingelfinger; Pleural Effusion, a review, N Engl J Med 2018;378:740-51.

parapneumonic effusion or it can become infected and become an *empyema*. Less common causes of exudates include infection with the tuberculosis organism, a pulmonary embolism or infarct, cancer, intraabdominal infections, and autoimmune diseases.

The most common symptom of a pleural effusion is pain. If the effusion involves inflammation of the parietal pleura, the patient will have "pleurisy" or a pleuritic chest pain. The patient has pain when he or she breathes. He or she will grab his or her chest when taking a deep breath. A less common chest discomfort occurs with large effusions. The patient may have a feeling of fullness in the chest.

The second symptom, which is less commonly seen, is shortness of breath, which may be due in part to atelectasis caused by compression of the lung by the fluid. Lastly, cough is occasionally seen as well. The cough is typically a dry cough and may be related to underlying atelectasis caused by the compression of the lung by the pleural effusion.

Trepopnea is a form of positional dyspnea in which the patient has **less** shortness of breath when he lies on the side with the pleural effusion. Likely it is due to better matching of ventilation and perfusion when the patient lies in that position.

The physical exam shows dullness and decreased breath sounds over the pleural fluid. Importantly, the trachea and heart should be shifted away from the fluid. If they are shifted towards the side of the effusion, atelectasis must also be present as well as the effusion. The location of the trachea is easy to find. Just place your index finger in the suprasternal space. The trachea should be directly in the middle of the space. The position of the heart also can be readily determined, either by percussion of the left heart border or by feeling the apical pulse, which should be in the mid-clavicular line at about the 5th interspace on the left.

Some patients, especially those with an inflammatory pleural lesion will have a pleural friction rub which sounds like "two pieces of leather being rubbed together." The sound is dramatic when you hear it.

Pulmonary function testing shows a restrictive pattern in patients with at least a moderate effusion. When the fluid is removed the pulmonary function may improve significantly.

The diagnosis of a pleural effusion is usually made by a chest radiograph. Free pleural fluid is always dependent. If the patient is standing the fluid is in the lower part of the chest. If the patient lies on his left side, the fluid will be along the left lateral chest wall. If, however, the fluid is *loculated*, or "trapped," the fluid will not change position with a change in the position of the patient.

There are additional findings to suggest that a localized opacity on the chest radiograph is an effusion and not a pneumonia or atelectasis. The most important is the presence of the *meniscus sign*. Free-flowing pleural effusions will appear to "climb up" the lateral wall of the chest. It is similar to the reaction that water has with the sides of a glass. Put water in a glass and then look at the sides of the glass. The water appears to climb up the sides of the glass. This is due to the relatively charged water (water has a positive side made up of the two hydrogen ions and a negative side made up of the one oxygen molecule) and the silicon dioxide molecules of the glass. The molecules attract each other, and the water climbs the side of the glass.

One important clue to the etiology of a pleural effusion based on the chest x-ray alone is whether there is a shift in the heart shadow and mediastinum. With a moderate pleural effusion, the heart shadow and mediastinum should be shifted away from the effusion. If the pleural fluid is on the left side, the heart should be pushed to the right. If it is not, then there must be significant atelectasis on the side of the effusion. This is almost always caused by cancer causing both the atelectasis and the effusion.

If the chest radiograph confirms the presence of a pleural effusion then, unless the patient has an obvious cause for the effusion such as congestive heart failure, the fluid should be sampled. The procedure is called a thoracentesis. A small needle is inserted, using an ultrasound for guidance, through the skin, directed above the rib (in order to avoid the nerves and blood vessels that run under the rib, into the pleural space. As the needle passes through the parietal pleura the patient will feel a sharp pain for an instant. The fluid is then sampled using a syringe or drained using an underwater seal.

Several studies on the fluid can be done. Protein, LDH, cell count, and glucose are routinely measured. Smears and cultures are sent for gram stain and culture, and an AFB smear and culture are sent looking for tuberculosis. A sample is also sent for cytology. Cytology is the study of the appearance of the cells in the fluid and is done in order to see if any cancer cells are present.

The protein and LDH are used to determine if the fluid is a transudate or an exudate. Transudates have little protein and LDH. To be a transudate the pleural fluid must meet two major criteria. First, the ratio of the pleural fluid protein to blood protein level must be less than 0.5. In other words, if the blood protein is 6 gms/100 ccs, the pleural fluid protein must be less than 3 gms/100 ccs. Secondly, the ratio of the pleural fluid LDH to the blood LDH must be less than 0.6. For example, if the serum LDH is 100 then the pleural fluid LDH must be less than 60.

Sometimes the level of cholesterol in the fluid is also measured to help differentiate a transudate from an exudate when the LDH and protein studies are not consistent with each other.

The glucose is measured because certain types of fluid, usually those with an abundance of inflammatory cells or with cancer cells, will have low sugar. Cancer involving the pleural space, an empyema, tuberculosis, or rheumatoid arthritis can cause a low sugar. The cell count is studied to determine whether there are a lot of neutrophils suggesting an infection such as an empyema. A lot of eosinophils suggest the presence of air or blood in the pleural space. An abundance of lymphocytes suggests the patient may have either tuberculosis or a lymphoma, which is a cancer of the lymph nodes. If an empyema is suspected a pH is done as well. The pH will be low in fluid caused by empyema, tuberculosis, or an esophageal rupture.

In the presence of an empyema the gram stain will usually show the causative organism, whether it is gram positive, like S. pneumoniae or St. aureus, or gram negative like Ps. aeruginosa or E. coli. Culture the fluid will generally identify the causative organism. The key findings of an empyema are the presence of an exudate with a low sugar and a low pH as well as a positive gram stain and culture.

The treatment of a pleural effusion should always be directed at its underlying cause. If the fluid is due to an empyema, the fluid must be drained, and the drain must be left in place until there is no further drainage. An empyema is like an abscess on your skin. It will not heal with antibiotics alone. You must drain the abscess to allow healing to take place. Thus an empyema requires a larger chest tube placed into the pleural space as well as antibiotics. Sometimes the empyema is composed of pockets of pus and surgery must be done to break up the pockets to allow adequate drainage. Once the infection is controlled the tube can be removed.

If the effusion is very large and the patient is short of breath, then the fluid should be removed in total. If the patient's shortness of breath is improved, just like in the case of an empyema, a tube should be inserted to keep the fluid drained until the patient is better.

Sometimes, tube drainage is not enough. The fluid just drains and drains. If the fluid is benign (not due to cancer), a *pleurodesis* can be done. A pleurodesis involves draining the fluid from the chest cavity using a large bore tubing connected to an underwater seal and then instilling an irritating chemical such as talc, tetracycline, or bleomycin (an anticancer medication) into the chest cavity. The tube is closed for several hours to allow the medicines to work. Then, the tube is opened to drainage. Hopefully over the next couple of days the effusion will abate.

A different approach is used if the patient does not respond to pleurodesis or if the patient has cancer. A small tube, called a *pigtail catheter*, is placed through the skin into the pleural space in order to drain the chest cavity. The pigtail has a one-way valve and a small reservoir which can be drained as needed. This allows the patient to go home and spend some time with his family and friends.

A **hemothorax** is the presence of blood in the pleural space. This is most often due to trauma, but cancer, renal failure, or tuberculosis can be the culprit as well. The blood should almost always be drained. Failure to remove the blood can result in a "trapped lung" or "orange peel lung" in which the lung develops a thick fibrous coating around it resulting in restrictive disease. The "peel" has to be removed surgically and the surgical procedure is, as you might imagine, quite bloody.

A **pneumothorax** is defined as air in the pleural space. It can be caused by either:

1. Direct damage to the lung resulting in a hole in the visceral pleura:
    a. "Secondary spontaneous pneumothorax" is the rupture of a bleb or bulla in a patient with emphysema or in a patient with HIV and a Pneumocystis jiroveci infection. However, a pneumothorax can also occur spontaneously in tall, thin, otherwise healthy young (generally early twenties), men who have tiny blebs at the top of their lungs. This is called a "primary

spontaneous pneumothorax." Most of these young men are smokers. The disorder appears to be genetic though the inheritance pattern is unclear as of the moment.

    b. Chest wall trauma such as a fractured rib tearing the lung and causing an air leak.

    c. Placement of a Swan-Ganz catheter via the subclavian artery. This procedure is done blindly. The needle is placed under the clavicle and above the underlying rib. Occasionally the underlying lung can be torn. A chest radiograph must always be done after the placement of a Swan-Ganz catheter via this approach to be sure there is no pneumothorax.

    d. Positive pressure ventilation can also cause a tear in the lung. This is unlikely to occur if the peak pressure is less than 25 mm Hg but once that threshold is exceeded the risk increases linearly. A peak pressure of 50 mm Hg results in a 50% chance of a pneumothorax.

2. Break in the chest wall resulting in a tear in the parietal pleura:
    a. Chest wall trauma such as a knife or gunshot wound resulting in a penetrating or open wound.

The symptoms of a pneumothorax are quite variable. A small amount of air in the pleural space will likely be asymptomatic while a large amount of air, such as when a patient with emphysema blows out a bulla in his lung completely collapsing the lung, will be quite symptomatic. The latter patient will have severe shortness of breath. In addition, patients with primary spontaneous pneumothorax usually present with chest pain.

There is one type of pneumothorax which is always life-threatening. This is the *tension pneumothorax*. In this circumstance the tear in the lungs behaves as a "one-way valve." Air leaks from the lung into the pleural space during inspiration as the chest expands and the pressure in the pleural space falls, but during exhalation the leak closes, trapping the air in the pleural space. The air in the pleural space increases rapidly, pushing the heart, great vessels, and trachea away from the side with the collapsed lung. Ultimately, this will cause circulatory collapse and a true medical emergency. The physician or emergency technician must be suspicious of this calamity. If a patient has chest wall trauma with the presence of subcutaneous air or "crepitus," which feels a little like Kellogg's Post Krispies under the skin, as well as tracheal deviation to the side away from the injury, then a tension pneumothorax is very likely. A penknife or other handy penetrating object must be thrust into the damaged chest to save the day.

A tension pneumothorax is even more likely to occur in the ICU. Typically, a patient on positive pressure ventilation will suddenly develop increased dyspnea while the peak ventilator pressure climbs abruptly and the SaO2 falls dramatically. This is either due to a mucous plug in an airway or to a pneumothorax. If it is a pneumothorax, because of the positive pressure ventilation, it is almost always a tension pneumothorax. The only exception would be if the patient has a chest tube already in place.

Physical findings of a pneumothorax are quite variable. If the pneumothorax is small, the examination will be normal. If it is large, then the involved hemithorax will be a bit larger than the normal hemithorax and will have a tympanic percussion note. Breath sounds will be diminished. These findings will be exaggerated if the patient has a tension pneumothorax. As with a pleural effusion, the trachea will be shifted away from the side of the pneumothorax. This is easily evaluated by placing the index finger in the suprasternal notch. The trachea should normally be midline. As with a pleural effusion, the apex of the heart, which is generally quite palpable in the fourth or fifth interspace in the midclavicular line, will also be shifted away from the side with the pneumothorax.

The diagnosis is generally made by the chest radiograph. As the lung collapses it becomes denser and appears greyer on the chest x-ray. There is generally a thin even greyer line outlining the collapsed lung. Outside of the collapsed lung, the space is black, devoid of any blood vessels. In a patient with COPD and a small pneumothorax, a CAT scan may be needed to make the diagnosis. Students often look first for the gray line outlining the collapsed lobe or lung. This line is often very difficult to see. It is far easier to look for the gray collapsed lobe or lung first.

Treatment largely depends on the size of the pneumothorax. If it is small, then just giving oxygen and observation will be enough. When oxygen is given, the pO2 in the blood and tissue surrounding the pneumothorax increase resulting in a compensatory fall of the nitrogen concentration. The gradient between the nitrogen in the air inside the pneumothorax and the surrounding tissue is increased, hastening absorption of the air. Because oxygen is consumed by the tissue the gradient for oxygen is not affected.

If the pneumothorax is more than 20% of the hemithorax, then the air should be removed by placing a pigtail catheter with a one-way valve into the chest cavity, allowing the air to leave. If it is a tension pneumothorax, immediate drainage must be done with anything handy.

Occasionally, the patient will have a combination of a pleural effusion and pneumothorax. The easiest way to make the diagnosis of a "hydropneumothorax" is to look for the meniscus sign along the lateral chest wall. There won't be one. The treatment is the same as for an uncomplicated pneumothorax.

The patient with primary or secondary spontaneous pneumothorax has a significant risk of having a second pneumothorax. In fact, the risk is about 25%. If a second pneumothorax occurs, then there is a 50% risk of a third. Most patients who have had two pneumothoraces should have either a chemical pleurodesis or a mechanical pleurodesis done via thoracoscopy.

Mesotheliomas are tumors of the mesothelial tissues. The mesothelium are thin tissues that envelope the lung, the heart and even the testicles, as well as provide the lining of the thorax and abdomen. In the chest wall, the mesothelium is called the pleura while in the abdomen it is the peritoneum.

All mesotheliomas are malignant. Most (75%) of mesotheliomas arise in the chest cavity. Peritoneal mesotheliomas account for most of the remaining cancers. Pericardial and testicular mesotheliomas are rare. There are two types of tumors, *epithelial* and *sarcomatoid* or *fibrous*.

There are about 3000 cases of mesothelioma a year. The tumor was rare before the 1970's, increasing in incidence until the 1990's and leveling off since then. Most cases are found in Caucasian and Hispanic men in the seventies.

The chance of surviving five years with the tumor is about 9%, but if the tumor is found early before it has spread to the lymph nodes or other tissue the chance of surviving five years is twice that.

Asbestos causes more than ninety percent of mesotheliomas both pleural and peritoneal. Peritoneal mesotheliomas are due to swallowing asbestos fibers. Less common causes include exposure to high dose radiation or to chemicals similar to asbestos. One such chemical is erionite which is found in rocks in Turkey.

The main symptom of a pleural mesothelioma is pain, most often pain due to involvement of the nerves of parietal pleura itself or to involvement of adjacent boney structures. If the tumor is in the upper lobes, the nerves to the arms and hands can be involved and the patient may present with arm or hand pain. The mesothelioma may cause a pleural effusion which can be quite large and may cause shortness of breath and cough.

Evaluation of the patient includes a chest radiograph and CAT scan. A PET scan (positron emission tomography scan) is helpful in distinguishing whether a pleural lesion is malignant or benign. It can also identify metastatic lesions. Two blood tests which are quite high in patients with mesotheliomas are the FIbulin-3 and the soluble mesothelin-related peptides (SMRPs). By themselves, the tests are NOT diagnostic, however. The diagnosis is made by biopsy or, if there is a pleural effusion, by studying the cells in the fluid. Treatment of the tumor is by surgery, radiation or chemotherapy including immunotherapy.

Suggestions for minor papers

1. What other options could Julius have had instead of the "tunneling procedure?"
2. What are treatment options for "flail chest?"
3. How does a tension pneumothorax cause cardiovascular collapse?
4. Compare the different causative mechanisms of a pleural effusion.
5. Compare primary and secondary spontaneous pneumothorax.
6. What is a pneumomediastinum and how is it related to a pneumothorax?
7. What is immunotherapy? What types of immunotherapy are available?

Eleven

Cystic Fibrosis

Cystic Fibrosis (CF) is the most common lethal inherited disease affecting Caucasians. It is an autosomal recessive disorder. Both parents must have at least one copy of the gene in order for the newborn to get the disease. About 1 in every 25 Caucasians are carriers, each having a normal gene and a gene for CF. Thus, one in every 2,500 live births among Caucasians result in a child with Cystic Fibrosis. But in some Caucasian subcultures the frequency of being a carrier is as high as one in twenty. There are one thousand cases of CF diagnosed every year in the United States, with about 30,000 people with CF currently alive in the United States. Worldwide there are about 70,000 cases. At first glance this sounds crazy. How come there are so many in the US compared to the whole world? It is because half of the world's Caucasian population resides in the US. But, Caucasians make up less than 1/7th of the world population.

In contrast, the incidence of CF among Hispanics is only about one in 9,500, among Blacks 1 in 15,000, and among Asians 1 in 31,000. But, Asians make up nearly half of the world's people.

Cystic fibrosis is a disease involving Chromosome 7. More than 70% of the time the mutation is Phe508del, the gene for phenylalanine. This amino acid is important for the folding the protein that forms the backbone of the chloride channel (CFTR or Cystic Fibrosis Transmembrane Conductase Regulator) correctly. If CFTR is not folded correctly it will be non-functional and the chloride ion cannot move in or out of the cell.

Because of the abnormal channel, the mucous of exocrine secreting tissues such as the glands of the lung or the glands of the pancreas becomes thick causing a blockage of ducts. This results in inflammation and ultimately scarring and destruction of the glands.

Over the last two decades treatment of CF has improved. Survival has gone from a life expectancy of only 20 years, when I was in medical school, to a life expectancy of more than 47 years. To a large measure this is due to the more effective use of respiratory therapy techniques though new types of medications have also been helpful.

Peter A. Petroff, MD

Case Presentations

1.

We are asked to see a twelve-year-old male, Michael, who is accompanied by his mother. The mother states her child has been ill for about a week with a severe cough productive of rust colored phlegm, associated with a spiking temperature and chills and right sided chest wall pain that hurts every time he takes a breath.

He was diagnosed with Cystic Fibrosis shortly after birth. He did not have his first bowel movement for more than 24 hours after delivery. A blood test was done which showed that he had CF. The mother believes the test was the "Immunoreactive Trypsinogen" test. The test was repeated twice and was positive both times. In addition, Michael went to the Cystic Fibrosis Foundation Clinic and had a sweat test when he was three years old which was positive for Cystic Fibrosis.

Despite the diagnosis of CF, Michael did well. He only had two or three upper respiratory illnesses a year and most were quite mild. His mother states he has colds no more often than his brother and sister. His appetite is good. His height and weight are normal for his age.

A year ago, however, Michael was hospitalized for five days with pneumonia. It was his first and only hospitalization. Since then, he has been on postural drainage and percussion, albuterol via a nebulizer four times a day, inhaled Dornase alfa, a multivitamin, and pancreatic enzymes. He does not have diabetes and has not had any other bowel disorder.

He regularly visits the CF clinic and has pulmonary function testing about twice a year. Surprisingly, they were normal. He has not had a chest x-ray in the past year.

When he was in the hospital last year, the patient in the bed next to him had a cardiac arrest and died. Michael looks at the doctor and says, "I don't ever want to go to the hospital."

Michael does not smoke or use any other medicine than his treatment for CF. He has no drug allergies. Both his parents are carriers. They have chosen not to have any more children. His brother is a carrier as well.

The doctor examines the young boy. His lips are bluish. He appears to be breathing faster than normal. He is diaphoretic. His blood pressure is 100/64; his pulse is 104; his temperature is 101.4. He has an obvious productive cough. The phlegm is rust colored. He has audible wheezes

Examination of his head and neck shows bilateral nasal polyps.

Examination of his lungs shows poor lung expansion. There is tactile fremitus over the right lower lobe. Auscultation reveals coarse crackles throughout the lungs but fine inspiratory crackles over the right lower lobe.

The rest of the exam is normal.

The doctor orders a chest radiograph, ABGs, CBC, a chemistry panel as well as sputum smear and cultures.

The patient refuses the ABGs. His O2 saturation is only 88% on room air. The Chest x-ray shows a right lower lobe pneumonia. The lungs are otherwise clear. The white count is high at 12,500 with increased neutrophils. The chemistry panel including the liver tests and albumin is normal.

After reviewing the results with Michael and his mother, the doctor advises the mother that Michael needs to be admitted to hospital. Reluctantly both Michael and his mother agree. A consultation is ordered for the social worker and Michael is admitted to a private room.

The doctor begins Michael on O2 at 2l/min by nasal cannula. His O2 saturation increases to 94%. He is started on intravenous fluids as well. The aerosol therapy with albuterol is continued and will be given every four hours. His Dornase, multivitamins, and pancreatic enzymes are also continued. The doctor begins Michael on Intravenous Amoxicillin (the dose is adjusted to his weight) as well as a fitted "inCourage Clearance Therapy" vest.

On the second day, the sputum Gram stain shows gram positive cocci in pairs and the cultures grows Streptococcus pneumoniae. The pneumococcus is sensitive to penicillin; the doctor continues the Amoxicillin.

On the third day Michael is much better. The oxygen is tapered; the antibiotic is switched to an oral form. He goes home the next day. He will continue the antibiotic for one more day and continue to use "the vest" as well as his postural drainage and aerosol therapy, and his other medications.

2.

Kathy is a 35-year-old woman who is being evaluated at the outpatient clinic because of severe sinusitis associated with increasing cough and purulent phlegm.

She tells the doctor she has had sinus problems since she was twenty and has seen several allergists. She was told she is allergic to cats and cedar as well as several foods. She got rid of her cats and avoided the offending foods. Those measures seemed to help for a while but in the last two or three years the symptoms have been persistent and worsening. She had a sinus drainage procedure a year ago which did not help at all. Last year she was treated for pneumonia.

She has coughed up a couple of ounces of yellow to green colored phlegm every day for the last six months. Occasionally, she has coughed up flecks of blood. She is short of breath walking more than one block. She has to take the elevator to the second floor at work because she can't walk up one flight of stairs. She has not had any fever or chest pain.

Her past history is important. She has never smoked nor lived with a smoker. She does not drink. She does not take any medicines and is not allergic to any medications that she knows of. Her only surgery has been sinus surgery. Her parents are dead. Her father had a heart attack at fifty and her mother died with influenza shortly after she was born. She has a history of headaches and malaise but has no history of arthritis or rash or gastrointestinal symptoms. She has no history of diabetes, but her sugars have been "a bit high" recently.

The doctor examines Kathy and notes the following: height is 165 cm with a weight of 64 kg resulting in a body mass index (BMI) of 23.5. She is afebrile, with an O2 saturation of 99%; there are no signs of respiratory distress. She has large nasal polyps bilaterally with tenderness over the right maxillary sinus, mild wheezing which clears with coughing, but persistent coarse crackles over both lung fields. Her abdominal exam is unremarkable. There is early clubbing bilaterally.

He orders several laboratory exams, including a chest radiograph, sinus x-rays, pulmonary function testing, sputum smear and culture including a culture for tuberculosis, as well as blood tests for IgE, alpha-1-antitrypsin, a CBC, and chemistry panel.

The PFTs show an FEV1 of 80% of predicted, an FVC of 81% of predicted, a normal FEV1/FVC ratio as well as normal diffusion capacity. The RV/TLC ratio was increased. The CXR showed changes consistent with mild bronchiectasis with "tram tracks" over both upper lobes. The sinus x-rays showed acute right maxillary sinusitis. The sputum grew Pseudomonas aeruginosa and the AFB smear for tuberculosis was 4+ positive. The culture for tuberculosis is still pending.

After reviewing the Chest radiograph with Kathy, the doctor ordered a High Resolution CAT scan of her lungs. He had originally planned to begin her on Levaquin, a fluoroquinolone, but when he saw the results of the AFB smear, he felt he had to wait till he got the nucleic acid amplification test for tuberculosis back before starting an antibiotic. The test should be back the next day.

The HRCAT scan of the chest showed severe bronchiectasis involving all the areas of the lung. There was mucous plug, tram lines, tree-in-bud opacities, as well as small fluid filled cavities and signet rings. The nucleic acid amplification test showed that the acid-fast organism was not Mycoplasma tuberculosis, the cause of tuberculosis. Thus, it must be an atypical Mycobacterium. They would have to wait for the culture and sensitivities.

He began the patient on Amoxicillin by mouth, aerosol therapy with a hand-held device, a nasally inhaled steroids for her sinusitis, and an orally inhaled steroid for her bronchiectasis. He ordered a sweat test as well.

The sweat test was indeterminate for cystic fibrosis.

Because Kathy had both an indeterminate sweat test and bronchiectasis, the doctor ordered genetic studies which showed that she had two abnormal genes for cystic fibrosis. The genes were not the types associated with severe disease.

Kathy returned after taking a ten-day course of the antibiotic. She was much better. The doctor told her she likely had cystic fibrosis and he discussed several treatments that should be begun at once. He began her on Dornase alfa and an Albuterol inhaler. He also demonstrated the use of a "flutter valve" and gave her one to try at home. He told her she should have a chest radiograph every year and pulmonary function testing twice a year. She must also check her sugars frequently, at least once a week.

He saw her back again in one month. She continued to improve. The sputum grew M. avium as expected. Based on the sensitivity study, the doctor began her on four medications to which the organism was sensitive. She would need to take the medications for at least one year.

He saw her again in a month. The cough had gone away, and she had gained a little weight. Even the shortness of breath was better.

3.

Alfredo Z. is a 31-year-old man, who was diagnosed with cystic fibrosis at the age of 6 months. He has done well though his pulmonary function testing has deteriorated over the last two years, and he was hospitalized 6 months ago with respiratory failure. He was treated in the ICU with non-invasive ventilation. The hospital course was stormy, but he survived. He is referred to the Cystic Fibrosis Lung Transplantation Clinic.

The doctor reviews Alfredo's past history with him. Alfredo states he was diagnosed with cystic fibrosis shortly after birth. His Immunoreactive Trypsinogen test, repeated twice, was positive on both occasions. He was referred at six months to the Cystic Fibrosis Foundation. His sweat test was positive. He did well until he was three years old when he developed wheezing and cough. He was treated with an inhaler, which he still takes. At age 12, he had his first bout of pneumonia. Since then, he has had more than a dozen attacks of pneumonia. When he turned sixteen, he developed diabetes and has been on insulin since then. His pulmonary function studies at age 20 were:

Test	% of predicted
FEV1	75%
FVC	100%
MMF	60%
TLC	123%
RV	120%
Diffusion	90%

The doctor at the CF clinic began him on Dornase alfa daily, inhaled Tobi (tobramycin) twice a day, an Albuterol inhaler, a high frequency oscillating chest wall device, and azithromycin 250 mg three times a week as well as hypertonic saline. The doctor continued the pancreatic enzyme replacement as well as fat soluble vitamins. The insulin was continued as well.

Alfredo states that he did quite well. At the age of 24, he married a CF negative young woman who he adores and fathered two children even though he had azoospermia due to obstruction of the vas deferens. This was accomplished using microsurgical epididymal sperm aspiration followed by in vitro fertilization. He adores his children dearly. He worked in management and rose steadily in the corporation. He states that he did not have the time to go back to the clinic twice a year. Finally, at the age of 28, he returned to his doctor. He was much shorter of breath, his cough was worse, and he was worried about his children. The doctor was concerned. He ordered pulmonary function studies:

Test	% of predicted
FEV1	45%
FVC	62%
MMF	25%
TLC	139%
RV	130%
Diffusion	85%

Alfredo had stopped his Tobi, hypertonic saline and Zithromycin. He rarely used his "vest." "I just didn't have the time to mess with all that stuff." But now he agreed he would "do everything I am supposed to do." The doctor ordered a sputum culture and sputum for AFB. He also did routine laboratories including checks on Alfredo's diabetes and his sodium and potassium as well as his liver and kidneys. All his treatments were resumed.

The doctor saw him again in six months. Alfredo felt better with less cough and dyspnea. However, the pulmonary function was worse.

Test	% of predicted
FEV1	35%
FVC	45%
MMF	20%
TLC	130%
RV	130%
Diffusion	75%

The doctor was quite concerned. Alfredo was taking his medications regularly but was steadily getting worse. The sputum culture grew Pseudomonas aeruginosa as expected. Burkholderia cepacia was not found, which was a very happy finding as it is an extremely resistant bacterium. Nor was there any growth of a Mycobacterium or a fungus such as Aspergillosis.

Six months ago, Alfredo developed fever, chills, a severe bloody cough, and shortness of breath. He was admitted to hospital and placed in the ICU. He was treated with IV tobramycin as well as Ceftazidime, a third-generation cephalosporin, and Vancomycin. He was placed on non-invasive ventilation and oxygen. Miraculously, he did not have to be intubated. After a difficult course spanning three weeks in the hospital, he was discharged home on his regular medication as well as cefdinir and oxygen at two liters per minute via a cannula. He was in rehabilitation for a month and then went back to work part time. He saw his doctor after he completed the rehabilitation. The doctor checked his chest radiograph, oxygen saturation and his pulmonary function. He told Alfredo that his FEV1 was 28% of predicted, "Alfredo, it's time you see the transplant clinic." Alfredo told the doctor, "I need to talk with my wife and family."

Finally, as his breathing worsened, Alfredo made the decision to see the transplant clinic. The doctor discussed with Alfredo and his wife what a transplant entails, "The hardest part is the wait. Nowadays, the success rate is great. If you make it past the first year without problems, your new lung should last an average of ten years." He went on, "You meet all the requirements for a transplant. We need to get a bunch of tests as soon as possible, and if they are ok, we will put you on the list."

The testing was extensive and included several heart studies and bone density testing in addition to the pulmonary tests. His sputum was still free of Burkholderia cepacia. Alfredo was placed on the waiting list. Two weeks later, at 2 AM, he got the call. He went at once to the University Hospital. His wife took the children to stay with her grandmother. On arrival at the emergency room, Alfredo was taken to the preoperative surgical suite where he met the anesthesiologist and surgeon. The new lungs would arrive within an hour. An IV was inserted and tests including blood gases were done. He was begun on Voriconazole, an antifungal agent used to treat Aspergillosis.

Alfredo's wife arrived just before he was taken to surgery. The surgery lasted six hours. After surgery he was admitted to the ICU on a ventilator. The settings were A/C of 12, TV of 400 cc, 5 cm PEEP, and 50% oxygen. The doctor wanted to keep him intubated for 6 hours.

At six hours, a chest radiograph and blood gases were done. The chest x-ray showed a minimal but definite interstitial infiltrate throughout all the lung fields. The blood gases had been done on 100% oxygen. The pO2 was only 250. Thus, the PaO2/fiO2 ratio was 250 indicating mild ARDS. The doctor checked Alfredo's wedge pressure. It was 18. He ordered Lasix and said he would check the chest radiograph in the morning. Alfredo was returned to 40% oxygen.

The next morning, Alfredo was again place on 100% oxygen and a chest radiograph was done. The x-ray was now clear and the PaO2 was 550, which was normal. The sedation was stopped. After an hour, Alfredo was placed on a T piece at 28%. One hour later blood gases were again done. The doctor then extubated Alfredo.

Three days later, he was discharged to undergo rehabilitation. The day of discharge, Alfredo told the doctor, "I can really breathe. My cough is gone. I don't need oxygen. I have been reborn."

He was discharged on the Voriconazole, Ganciclovir for Cytomegalovirus, Cyclosporine, Prednisone, and mycophenolic acid. The last three agents are used for immunosuppression to prevent rejection of the new lungs. All the medications for CF were stopped except for his pancreatic replacement enzymes and his vitamins. He also continued his insulin.

After two weeks he went back to work. His coworkers could not believe how great he looked. After three months he returned to the clinic for a bronchoscopy with a lung biopsy as well as a chest radiograph. The biopsy showed no evidence of rejection. The sputum showed only a light growth of pseudomonas. He would need to take the antirejection drugs for the rest of his life and would have to have a bronchoscopy every three months. He told the doctor, "It's all worth it."

Peter A. Petroff, MD

Background for the Presentation

These three cases illustrate the enormous spectrum of cystic fibrosis. In the first case we have a young man who was diagnosed with cystic fibrosis at birth. In the second case we have a woman who was not diagnosed with CF until she was in her mid-thirties. Michael presented with mild though persistent symptoms of cough and phlegm but with typical pneumonia. Kathy presented with a one-year history of sinusitis and was found to have bronchiectasis on her chest radiograph. Both patients have significant though different findings important to both the diagnosis and the treatment of the disease. Alfredo, the third cased study, is a patient who, having had CF for thirty years, finally comes to a lung transplant.

Important Points.

1. Cystic fibrosis is a multisystem disease. The two most important target organs that cystic fibrosis affects are the lungs and the pancreas.
2. C.F. has an autosomal recessive inheritance.
3. The underlying defect is in the CFTR protein which operates the intracellular chloride channel.
4. Pulmonary function testing generally reveals obstructive disease, at least early in the course.
5. The gold standard for diagnosis, especially in children, remains the sweat test. Other diagnostic tests include the IRT (Immunoreactive Trypsinogen), the nasal potential difference as well as genetic testing to identify the abnormality on chromosome 7.
6. Treatment relies strongly on intensive respiratory therapy including postural drainage and percussion and devices such as the "vest." A mucolytic agent such as Dornase alfa, an enzyme which breaks down DNA, has been shown to be helpful as well. The Cystic Foundation also recommends the use of inhaled hypertonic saline as well as nebulized antibiotics, such as tobramycin (Tobi). Bronchodilators such as Albuterol are likely helpful as well. Inhaled steroids such as Flovent are generally given but their use remains controversial. Pancreatic enzymes and multivitamins are needed to help prevent malabsorption and osteoporosis. Most patients with CF have diabetes by the time they turn twenty. The diabetes of cystic fibrosis is different from both type 1 and type 2 diabetes and requires insulin.
7. The newest medications work directly on the chloride channel and include ivacaftor, lumacaftor and vacaftor in combination, and Tezacaftor with ivacaftor in combination.
8. Lung transplantation has become an important therapy as well. It offers up to a ten-year survival. (The presenter for case 3 should discuss lung transplantation in detail, including indications, pre-operative testing, the surgery itself, and postoperative care.)

Discussion

Cystic Fibrosis likely has been a human disease for thousands of years. The earliest reference to the disease is in middle age folklore, "Woe is the child who tastes salty from a kiss on the brow, for he is cursed, and soon must die." By 1595, the relationship between salty skin and pancreatic disease was firmly established among doctors but it was not given a name until 1938 when Dr. Dorothy Andersen described children who died of malnutrition as having "cystic fibrosis of the pancreas." The disease also came to be known as "mucoviscidosis" because of the thick mucus associated with exocrine glands. Ten years later, Dr. Paul di Sant'Agnese observed infants suffering from severe dehydration during a New York heat wave. Based on his findings, he showed that the sweat of children with CF had abnormally high concentrations of salt thus validating the ancient folklore. In the early 1980's the protein responsible for the disease was found and in the late 1980's the genetic defect on chromosome 7 was discovered.

There are nearly two thousand different mutations on chromosome 7 that can cause cystic fibrosis. Because of this, the disease has protean manifestations from life-threatening, aggressive bronchiectasis to a disease that may not present until the patient is in their sixties. The most common mutation is at the site on the chromosome responsible for the manufacture of phenylalanine (phe508del), an amino acid that makes up part of the chloride channel and which is important in the proper folding of the protein.

The disease is an autosomal recessive disorder. This means the patient with CF must have two abnormal genes, one of which came from his or her father and one from his or her mother. Both his parents were either carriers of the disease, having one good gene and one bad gene or actually had CF and thus had two copies of the bad gene.

The chloride channel is regulated by CFTR protein and cyclic adenosine monophosphate or cAMP. The cAMP must attach to the CFTR protein for the chloride channel to operate. There are several genetic defects which can interfere with this reaction. The CFTR protein can be completely absent. The CFTR protein can be defective. The regulation by cAMP can be disordered by the inability of cAMP to bind to CFTR. All these aberrations will result in defective conductance of the chloride ion through the channel.

There are several classes of defects:

Class 1 mutations involve defective protein production.

Class 2 mutations involve defective protein processing which prevents the protein from moving to the correct cellular location. The gene involved is the phe508 del gene and is the most common mutation. 90% of all patients with cystic fibrosis will have at least one gene with this defect; half will have two genes with the defect.

Class 3 mutations involve defective regulation which will decrease the Chloride channel activity in response to ATP.

Class 4 mutations involve defective chloride conduction. In this defect, the protein is produced correctly, and it is correctly localized in the cell. In addition, unlike Class 3 mutations, the protein will respond to cAMP, but the rate of Chloride flow and the duration of channel opening are reduced.

Class 5 mutations involve a decreased amount of functional CFTR protein because the protein produced is not stable.

If the chloride ion cannot leave the cell, then sodium will transfer from outside the cell to inside the cell in order to maintain electrical neutrality dragging molecules of water with it. The surface of the cell will have less fluid resulting in mucus which is thicker and stickier to bacteria, causing colonization by bacteria and subsequent inflammation and infection. In addition, since the bicarbonate ion is also regulated by the CFTR protein, the HCO_3^- cannot be excreted and the area surrounding the cell will become acidotic. When the surface of the airway becomes acidotic, its ability to eliminate bacteria is impaired.

Cystic fibrosis affects mainly the lungs and the pancreas but any exocrine gland can be involved by the disease process. In order to make the diagnosis of cystic fibrosis, the patient must have a disease consistent with the diagnosis in at least one organ system and a positive sweat test or a DNA assay showing two mutations in the CFTR gene. **Cystic fibrosis (CFTR) related disease** is diagnosed when the clinical disease is limited to one organ and is associated with some evidence of CFTR dysfunction. Our second case fits into this category. This group includes patients with chronic sinusitis, chronic pancreatitis, azoospermia, or adult-onset pulmonary disease. Genetic testing may be needed to confirm the diagnosis in these patients.

Most patients with CF die of end-stage lung disease. At birth, the lungs of CF patients are normal. Shortly after birth the ducts of the submucosal glands become dilated. Then, the child develops a lung infection which causes a severe inflammatory response. The persistence of the inflammatory response allows the bacteria to colonize the airways and a cycle of recurrent infections begins. This results in the dilated bronchial tubes and bronchiectasis. Not surprisingly, second-hand smoke will accelerate the loss of lung function, especially in patients with the phe508del mutation.

The pancreas is largely responsible for the production, not just of insulin, but also of the enzymes which help us absorb our food including the lipases which break down fats and the proteinases which break down proteins into their component amino acids. In addition, the pancreas secretes HCO_3^- which neutralizes our stomach acid. These functions of the pancreas depend on the exocrine glands. CF causes the ducts of the exocrine glands to become blocked with debris resulting in inflammation and fibrosis of the pancreas.

Without the enzymes proteins and fat cannot be absorbed leading to "failure to thrive" in infants and progressive weight loss in teens and adults. The bacteria in the gut metabolize the fat resulting in the production of gas. Whatever fats are not absorbed pass through the bowels and result in foul-smelling fatty stools. In addition, the body cannot absorb the fat-soluble vitamins A, D, E, and

K. Vitamin D deficiency causes osteomalacia and Vitamin K deficiency can result in bleeding disorders. Vitamin E deficiency in infants can result in neurological impairment.

One of the early hallmarks of the disease is known as "meconium ileus." The meconium or stool of the newborn with CF has increased viscosity, decreased water content, and increased albumin making the stool thicker and more difficult to pass. The baby, unable to pass its stool, develops abdominal distension, vomiting and severe abdominal pain. Up until two decades ago, most physicians believed that meconium ileus was due to disease of the pancreas. Recent studies in mice have shown that meconium ileus is due to the involvement of the gut lining itself. Interestingly most children with CF do not have meconium ileus. They have no signs of CF till they are much older. Meconium ileus occurs in less than 10% of patients with CF and is much more frequently seen in children with the phe508del gene, especially if an additional genetic defect is present. This second defect is called a "modifier gene." Adults can have problems with their gut as well. Distal intestinal obstruction syndrome can occur which is characterized by a fecal mass at the ileocecal junction, abdominal distention with pain as well as vomiting. Other gastrointestinal complications include gastric reflux and recurrent pancreatitis.

Additional manifestations of CF include pansinusitis with nasal polyps and involvement of the ducts of the liver resulting in cirrhosis of the liver with all its consequences as well as gallstones and disease of the urogenital tract resulting in male sterility due to absence of the vas deferens and relative female infertility due to the presence of thick mucus filling the cervical canal.

The median age for the diagnosis of CF is six months. Half are diagnosed before six month and half afterwards. Two-thirds are diagnosed before their first birthday. The presentation varies with age. Neonates present with meconium ileus, young infants present with wheezing or coughing often due to pneumonia though some children present with failure to thrive and fatty stools. Later in childhood and into adulthood chronic cough is the main presenting feature. Some young children present with "steatorrhea," characterized by frequent, bulky, foul-smelling, and greasy stool that floats on the water in the commode.

The symptoms, signs, and disorders due to CF are protean and include:

1. Respiratory tract:
    a. Productive cough with thick yellow-green phlegm often with flecks of blood
    b. Shortness of breath
    c. Wheezing and atypical asthma
    d. Sinusitis and nasal polyps
    e. Bronchiectasis and even Allergic Bronchopulmonary Aspergillosis
    f. Pulmonary hypertension and cor pulmonale
2. Pancreatic disease:
    a. Steatorrhea
    b. Weight loss

    c. Anorexia (loss of appetite)
    d. Osteomalacia or Rickets due to Vitamin D deficiency (especially in females)
    e. Ultimately diabetes and its consequences may occur
3. Liver disease:
    a. Jaundice
    b. Abdominal pain due to gallstones
    c. Cirrhosis
4. Gastrointestinal tract:
    a. Meconium ileus
    b. Rectal prolapse
    c. Fatty stools
5. Urogenital disease:
    a. Undescended testis
    b. Hydrocele
    c. Male or female infertility
    d. Amenorrhea
6. Cutaneous:
    a. Salty tasting sweat
    b. Clubbing
    c. Dry skin due to vitamin A deficiency
    d. Cheilosis (painful swelling of the corners of the mouth) due to Vitamin B complex deficiency

The gold standard test for the diagnosis of CF is the sweat test or *quantitative pilocarpine iontophoresis test (QUIT)*. The sweat test takes advantage of the fact that sweat is produced by glands that are **not** dependent on the CFTR protein. In patients with CF, the sweat produced by the sweat glands cannot be reabsorbed because the epidermal cellular chloride channels are blocked. Sodium and chloride ions become trapped on the skin surface often forming crystals of salt. Thus, the infant has salty-tasting skin.

The QUIT is done by applying a small amount of pilocarpine, which stimulates sweat production, then applying a gentle electrical current to the site to activate the sweat glands. The sweat is collected. At least 50 mg of sweat is needed. The sweat is then analyzed for the chloride ion. The normal value is less than 30 mmol/l. Children with cystic fibrosis have values greater than 60 mmol/l. To be diagnostic in adults the level should exceed 80 mmol/l. The test **must** be confirmed with a second test.

False negatives can occur with low volumes of sweat, so the test is difficult to do in infants. False positives may also occur in conditions such as hypothyroidism, adrenal insufficiency, and malnutrition.

If the sweat test cannot be done, then the IRT or Immunoreactive Trypsinogen test should be done. This test is now done universally on all newborns in every state in the United States. This test must be confirmed by repeating the test, doing a DNA assay, or by doing a sweat test.

The nasal potential difference measures the potential difference in voltage from the nasal mucosa to the forearm. It correlates well with the movement of the sodium ion across cell membranes. Normally, sodium is excreted by the cell into the interstitial fluid but in patients with CF the movement is in the other direction. At the present time, because of the complicated equipment required for the test, this test is only available at research centers.

The last test is genotyping. This test is done only in patients with a family history of CF or in a couple who are planning to have a child. The test can detect more than 98% of Caucasian patients with a mutated gene. It is not as accurate in Asians, Hispanics, or Blacks.

Pulmonary Function testing must be done every six months to evaluate the severity of the pulmonary disease and its progress. Using the forced oscillation technique, the airway resistance can be measured even in infants. In older children and adults, the FEV1 is especially useful as it correlates directly with the progression of the disease. A chest radiograph should be done yearly. Sputum should be cultured annually.

Pseudomonas does not appear early in the course of the disease, but at about the age of twelve, the organism makes its appearance in the microbiome of the airway. Before it is in the microbiome it is treatable with inhaled tobramycin. Afterwards, it become persistent. Mycobacterium avium and Mycobacterium abscesses are also common pathogens. Recently, Burkholderia cepacia has become a major problem for the patient with CF. It is extremely resistant to antibiotics, and of more concern, it can be transferred from one CF patient to another CF patient. **Almost all, if not all, Cystic Foundation Clinics isolate patients with Burkholderia cepacia to prevent its spread**. Aspergillosis is also a common pathogen. It can cause Allergic Broncho-Pulmonary Aspergillosis. It can even be invasive causing a severe hemorrhagic, generally fatal, pneumonia.

The treatment of cystic fibrosis relies heavily on the respiratory therapist. Respiratory therapists are the cornerstones of therapy. But the treatment of CF must be a multidisciplinary approach including not only respiratory therapists and pulmonary physicians but also social workers, nutritionists and educators who are experienced with treating the disease and helping the family deal with the problems that surely will ensue. Because of that, therapy should best be given in a clinic or facility that is devoted to the treatment of cystic fibrosis. There are more than 120 centers in the United States that are supported and accredited by the Cystic Fibrosis Foundation.

The goals of therapy are three-fold. The first goal is to maintain lung function by preventing and aggressively treating infections. Secondly, it is imperative that the patient has good nutritional support. Malnutrition impairs the immune system increasing the risk of infection. Lastly, complications of the disease must be addressed early and thoroughly. All patients should have a DNA assay to determine the type of genetic defect that they have.

The mucus of patients with Cystic Fibrosis has a very high viscosity which is caused by the presence of glycoproteins, denatured DNA, and protein polymers such as actin. Treatment must be directed at these defects and at the present time includes:

1. Inhaled hypertonic saline:
   Several studies have shown that the FEV1 is improved with inhaled hypertonic saline which acts to thin mucous directly. Inhaled mannitol may sometimes be used instead.
2. Inhaled Dornase alfa:
   The airway becomes packed with white cells which break down over time releasing their DNA. DNA increases the viscosity of the mucous substantially. Dornase breaks the DNA down, improving lung clearance.
3. Inhaled bronchodilators such as albuterol:
   B adrenergic agents increase the mucociliary clearance by making the cilia beat stronger and faster.
4. Chest physical therapy including the use of high frequency chest wall compression therapy such as by the inCourage Airway Clearance System (the Vest). A flutter device may also be used as well as positive expiratory pressure
5. Nebulized antibiotics such as tobramycin (Tobi):
   Almost all, if not all, patients with CF are colonized with Pseudomonas infection. The sooner the inhaled Tobi is started the better. Ideally it should be started before the Pseudomonas becomes part of the biome of the airway.

The order of therapy, which is given twice a day is as follows: 1. Metered dose albuterol inhaler, 2. Hypertonic saline, 3. Dornase (once a day), 4. Chest physical therapy, 5. Aerosolized antibiotics. **Inhaled N-acetylcysteine (Mucomist) should not be used. It has not been shown to have clinical efficacy and may cause airway inflammation and bronchospasm.** Antimuscarinic agents have also been shown to have little benefit in patients with cystic fibrosis.

Other therapies include:

1. Low dose azithromycin:
   Azithromycin is an antibiotic, but it has anti-inflammatory properties as well. The use of the agent is controversial at the present time.
2. Pancreatic enzyme replacement therapy (PERT):
   All patients with CF need PERT.
3. Nutrition support including multivitamins:
   The fat-soluble vitamins, A, E, K and D need to be replaced. .Complications of not starting the vitamins include problems with vision,

problems with neurologic development, bleeding disorders and osteoporosis.
4. Anti-inflammatories such as inhaled steroids:
    Most consultants believe inhaled steroids should only be used in patients with asthma. However, 50% of patients with CF are using inhaled steroids while only about 15% of patients with CF are asthmatic.
5. Consideration should be given to the using the newest CFTR modulators: ivacaftor, lumacaftor/vacaftor and Tezacaftor/ivacaftor combinations:
    These CFTR modulators have recently been shown to be extremely effective, actually improving the FEV1 of patients. All patients over the age of six should have a DNA assay to determine what type of genetic mutation they have. If they have a phe508del mutation, they will likely respond to the new CFTR therapy. Therapy with Lumacaftor-ivacaftor is approved in children over the age of two. Tripple therapy is recommended in children over the age of six in patients with the phe508del mutation. Other mutations should be study in vitro before beginning the patient on the medicine to determine if there is a chance it will work.

Exacerbations should be treated swiftly with oral or intravenous antibiotics, increased frequency of chest physical therapy, and increased the dose of Pulmozyme (Dornase). Complications of CF include not only pneumonia and respiratory failure but also pneumothoraces.

Surgery can be considered as well and includes surgery for a collapsed lung, surgery for sinusitis, a partial pneumonectomy for severe localized disease and finally a lung transplant.

Lung transplantation is the ultimate therapy. As the survival of lung transplantations in patients with CF has improved and has more and more patients with CF lived into their thirties and forties, lung transplantation has been turned to more and more frequently. The average age of a lung transplant for CF is 30 with a slight male predominance.

16% of lung transplants are done in patients with CF. The median survival of a CF patient who has had a lung transplant is a little over 10 years. The overall five-year survival is 70% in one extensive series from the Toronto Lung Transplantation Program. 90% of patients who have had a lung transplant are satisfied. After they get their new lungs, their breathing is not just better, but it is nearly normal and, for most, their cough is completely gone.

The indications for a lung transplant in a patient with CF include an FEV1 of less than 30%, an oxygen saturation of less than 88%, an exacerbation of pulmonary disease requiring admission to the ICU, increased frequency of infections requiring antibiotics, refractory hemoptysis, and refractory pneumothorax. Contraindications include cancer in the last two years, HIV infection, certain infections with hepatitis B and C, and substance abuse within the last six months.

Before a person can be put on the transplant "waiting list" several tests must be done including a PFT, sinus and chest radiographs, arterial blood gases, ventilation/perfusion lung scan, CAT scan of the chest, abdominal ultrasound, CBC, chemistry profile (looks at kidneys and liver), MUGA scan, EKG, Thallium scan, and echocardiogram to evaluate heart status, bone mineral density, six-minute walk test, and sputum cultures.

Once on the waiting list, the patient must be ready to get to the hospital in a matter of minutes. They must live in close proximity to the hospital and always have a suitcase packed while they await the phone call or text that an organ is ready.

Some patients are already in hospital and are quite ill. These patients are usually placed on ECMO using a double lumen veno-veno system. The catheter is placed in the jugular vein and blood is taken from both the superior and inferior vena cava in returned to the right atrium. This allows the patient to be alert and able to exercise while awaiting the transplant. Using this system, the mortality of the waiting period has been cut nearly to zero!

Attention is also paid to the donor lungs. After the lung is removed it is also placed on a small ventilator and an ECMO type device. This keeps the donor lung healthier during the trip from one hospital where the organ was harvested to another where the organ will be implanted into the awaiting patient. Because the lung is ventilated, the risk of postoperative pulmonary edema is markedly reduced.

The surgery is long, taking anywhere from five to ten hours. The surgeon generally uses a clam shell approach. This allows the lungs to be removed one at a time. The most diseased lung is removed first, and a new lung implanted with attention to detail so that the bronchus, pulmonary artery, and bronchial arteries are all securely attached. While the lung is removed and the new lung implanted, the ET tube is placed in the contralateral lung to ventilate the patient. Then the same process is done on the other side. This way the patient does not need cardio-pulmonary bypass, decreasing the complication rate.

After surgery, the patient is taken to the ICU and allowed to awaken. Most patients are extubated in about 6 hours, but some do take longer. Primary Graft Dysfunction can occur in the first two or three days. It looks just like ARDS with hypoxemia and a ground glass appearance on the x-ray. Treatment is supportive with PEEP and lung protective ventilation. If the wedge pressure is increased, diuretics are used. Sometimes nitric oxide is used in more severe cases.

After discharge, the patient is sent home on immunosuppressive therapy, antifungal medicine, and a medicine to treat cytomegalovirus. Bactrim may be given to prevent Pneumocystis infection. They must be followed closely including bronchoscopies with biopsies, cultures and x-rays every three months.

Acute rejection of the new lung can occur anytime in the first year and is treated with high dose steroids. Late complications include bronchiolitis obliterans and pulmonary fibrosis.

The treatment of CF, especially with the CFTR regulators and lung transplantation is quickly evolving. A person born today with CF will likely live to be over 50!

Suggestions for Minor Papers

1. What different modalities can be used by the respiratory therapist in treating CF?
2. What order should the respiratory modalities be administered in?
3. What is the role of lung transplantation in CF?
4. How does hypertonic saline work? Why is it so highly recommended?
5. What other conditions are associated with nasal polyps?
6. What other conditions besides lung disease is associated with clubbing?
7. Describe the "clam-shell" surgical approach to lung transplantation?
8. Discuss why survival has changed so much in cystic fibrosis.
9. If you were a carrier for CF, would you have children? Why? Why not?
10. How is screening for CF done? How effective is screening?

References

1. Amy G. Filbrun, Thomas Lahiri, Clement L. Ren; Handbook of Cystic Fibrosis; Springer International Publishing Switzerland; 2016
2. Jonathan C. Yeung and Shaf Keshavjee; Overview of Clinical Lung Transplantation; Cold Springs Harbor Perspectives in Medicine, 2014; 4:ao15628
3. Song Yee Kim, Su Jin Jeong, et al.; Critical Care after Lung Transplantation; Acute and Critical Care; 2018 November 33 (4); 206-215
4. Jonathan C. Yeung, Tiago N. Machuca, Cecilia Chaparro, et. al; Lung Transplantation for Cystic Fibrosis; The Journal of Heart and Lung Transplantation; 2020; 39: 553-560 (Excellent summary of current status of lung transplantation from one of the largest transplant centers in the world)

Peter A. Petroff, MD

Twelve

Disorders of Sleep

We spend one third of our life sleeping. Why is sleep that important? It turns out sleep is necessary for two reasons. Firstly, sleep restores the chemicals in our brain necessary for us to function. Secondly, sleep is required for learning.

The neurons of the brain require cyclic-AMP (adenosine monophosphate) to function, but the metabolism of the brain is extremely limited. The cyclic AMP breaks down into adenosine which increases in brain tissue while we are awake. The brain is unable to convert it back to ATP. It is the buildup of adenosine which makes us sleepy. When we sleep, the adenosine is converted back into ATP and cyclic AMP so we will be ready for the next day.

Learning requires sleep. Rats who have been run a maze during the day will repeat and repeat running the maze at night and, after a good sleep, will run the maze much faster. Learning to play the piano or learning mathematics or memorizing for a test requires a good night's sleep.

But sleep is a problem for some people. They cannot fall asleep, or they cannot stay asleep. They have insomnia. Then there are people who are exactly the opposite. They cannot stay awake. Often it is because when they fall asleep, they cannot breathe because their airway is blocked, and they spontaneously awaken not once or twice an hour but sixty times an hour or even more. They just don't get a decent sleep. And it shows. They do not do well at school; they don't do well at work; they don't do well driving a car or an 18-wheeler. What's more they have often severe hypoxemia when they stop breathing which causes an inflammatory reaction resulting in the metabolic syndrome. Sleep disorders can cause hypertension, diabetes, and heart disease.

Still other patients are sleepy all the time because their brain confuses the sleeping and waking states. When these patients get excited, they go into REM sleep. Their body is paralyzed as if they are asleep, but their brain is still awake. This condition is fairly common, is often hereditable. It involves some families of Dachshunds and sheep as well as people and is called Narcolepsy.

Peter A. Petroff, MD

Case Presentations

1.

Howard C. is a 60-year-old truck driver. He comes to the internal medicine clinic because his wife says there's something wrong with him. She tells the doctor, "I can't take it anymore. He snores so loud; I have to sleep in the living room. He falls asleep watching TV, even the football games he says he has to watch. I refuse to get in the car if he is driving. He dosed off one time; we nearly hit a truck. I don't understand how he can drive his 18-wheeler."

Howard tells the doctor that his wife is exaggerating. He admits that he is a little sleepy. "I work long hours." He also says that he has gained a bit of weight. His wife shouts, "Forty pounds, doc!"

Howard never smoked. He does not drink. He sometimes takes medicines to keep him awake. Some of the medicines may be amphetamines he gets from fellow truck drivers. He has no drug allergies, surgeries, or medical admissions. He has not been to the doctor in more than fifteen years.

His examination shows him to be an obese male who appears his stated age. He is 5'10" tall and weighs 308 lbs. His blood pressure is 186/105. His pulse is 92. His SaO2 is 92% on room air. His neck circumference is 18 inches, and his weight circumference is 50 inches. He is afebrile.

The examination of the head and neck is unremarkable save for a large tongue. The neck veins are also slightly distended even with the head of the bed slightly elevated. The lungs are clear though breath sounds are a little decreased. The heart shows a grade 2/6 systolic murmur at the apex. There may be a soft third heart sound. The liver is enlarged to percussion and the liver edge is located 4 cm below the right costal margin. There is 2+ edema. The neurologic exam is normal.

The doctor asks the wife to step outside for a second. He turns off the lights in the room leaving Howard resting comfortably on the examination table. The doctor waits about 5 minutes. He and Mrs. C. return to the room, leaving the lights off. Howard is sound asleep. They watch as he stops breathing. Then, after what seems an eternity, his chest and abdomen begin to seesaw for a several seconds. Suddenly he snorts a ferocious snore. He sits up, he looks about. Then he lies down again. For a few seconds he breathes quietly. Then he stops breathing and the cycle repeats. The wife and doctor watch for about five minutes. Then the doctor rouses Howard.

"You have severe sleep apnea. We have to get some tests."

Howard confesses that he is not surprised. Some of his fellow truck drivers thought he had sleep apnea. The doctor orders fasting laboratory including a complete blood count, chemistry profile, hemoglobin A1C for diabetes, urinalysis, urine for microalbumin, EKG and a full sleep study. Howard asks why not get a home sleep study instead. The doctor says he has to be sure that Howard is sleeping; the home study does not look at the brain waves.

The complete blood count is normal. The chemistry panel shows the sugar to be 220. The kidney and liver tests are normal. The urine is normal but the test for microalbumin is positive. The EKG is normal. The sleep study is a split night sleep study. In the first half of the study Howard has an Apnea-Hypopnea Index of 60. With 14 cm of CPAP, the AHI becomes normal.

The doctor discusses the results with Howard and his wife. He begins Howard on Metformin 1500 mg with the evening meal for his diabetes as well as Vasotec and hydrochlorothiazide (a diuretic) for his high blood pressure. He discusses why these medicines are needed and what kind of bad things might occur if he does not take them. He also begins Howard on home CPAP. The doctor spends most of the time discussing lifestyle changes Howard needs to make and refers he and his wife to a nutritionist.

Howard returns two weeks later. He has lost more than twenty pounds. His blood pressure is normal. The edema is gone as is the heart murmur and third heart sound. In addition, his wife says he is sleeping soundly at night, and she is no longer afraid to let him drive her. The doctor orders a repeat fasting blood sugar which is 136.

Howard asks if he could stop the CPAP. The doctor says not right now but if Howard loses another twenty pounds, he will repeat the sleep study and see.

2.

Althea D. is a very pleasant young woman. She states, "I don't really know why I'm here. I must be crazy or something."

The doctor looks at her, "What do you mean?"

The young lady says, "I just seem to get "jelly legs" when I'm at a party."

She goes on to say that ever since she was in her early 20's she has been afraid to go out. If she went to a party and someone would tell a funny story or make a funny comment, her legs would get weak. One time she completely collapsed and fell. Thank heavens, she fell onto a sofa otherwise her friends might have had to pick her off the floor. Since that time, when she goes to a party or dance, she leans against the wall. If someone says something that might make her laugh, she gets weak but at least she does not fall. She does recall one very frightening episode which happened while she was watching TV. The program was really funny. She became totally weak. She couldn't even move her arms or legs or turn her head but, "You know what doctor. I could still hear the program. I couldn't move but I heard it all. The funnier it got, the harder it was for me to move."

She also notes that she has some daytime sleepiness, but it is generally pretty mild although she has to take a nap after school and sometimes even at lunch break. She feels good when she gets up in the morning. Lastly, she also had strange dreams when she falls asleep on occasion. "Sometimes they are pretty scary."

No one in her family ever had anything like that.

Her past history is unremarkable. She is thirty years of age. She does not smoke or drink. She takes no medications of any kind. She is not allergic to any medications. She has never been in a hospital and never had any surgery. She teaches high school English. She has taught English for more than ten years. "I've wanted to be a teacher since I was five years old."

She is a well-developed young woman in no acute distress. Her height is 5'4". She weighs 118 lbs. Her blood pressure is 104/60. Her pulse is 68. Her SaO2 is 96% on room air. She is afebrile.

Her examination is totally normal.

The doctor tells her he believes she has Narcolepsy, and that the weakness is a form of cataplexy. He advises her to get an overnight full polysomnogram and a multiple sleep latency test which will be done the following day.

The patient returns after the sleep study which showed a noticeably short sleep latency and early onset REM sleep. She definitely did not have sleep apnea. The multiple sleep latency test confirmed daytime sleepiness and early onset REM sleep. The doctor shows her the results. He says he is absolutely sure she has narcolepsy. He recommends she take two medications, one for daytime sleepiness and one for the "jelly legs." The first is a direct stimulant called Modafenil which she takes in the morning. If this does not improve the daytime sleepiness, then he would add a second medication called Sodium Oxybate which she should take twice at night. He also advises her to take a mild antidepressant, Prozac, for the "cataplexy." Lastly, he also advises her to continue her naps. "They are actually helpful."

Althea returned in two weeks. She is doing much better. She feels well. She continues her nap twice during the day and is taking her medications regularly. She feels much more secure at school. She no longer has to sit at her desk while she teaches. She feels safe enough to go out again.

3.

Rose N. is a pleasant 46-year-old woman who has been sent by her primary doctor to a sleep clinic "because I can't sleep." She tells the doctor, "All my life I have had trouble falling asleep. But it is getting worse and worse." She paused. "My husband says I sleep ok, but I know I don't."

The doctor asks her how she feels during the day. She says, "Oh, I'm a little tired but I get by."

She says she goes to bed at 9 PM and gets up at 7 AM. She says that it takes hours for her to fall asleep. She takes a sleeping pill, Ambien 5 mg, at bedtime. Sometimes she takes Benadryl as well. Her sister told her that a "hot toddy" will help so she takes an ounce of honey with a half-ounce of liquor just before bedtime. Her doctor has tried everything. "He even gave me an antidepressant called Trazadone. I walked around like a zombie for three days."

The doctor asks her, "Once you fall asleep do you stay asleep?"

"My husband says I sleep like a baby."

The doctor asks her about her bedroom. "Is there a TV? Is it dark? What's the temperature of the room?"

She says that she sometimes watches TV to "help me fall asleep." The room is dark although she has a tiny light near the bathroom door. The room is 78 degrees.

The doctor quizzes her about stress in her life. "I'm fine. I teach high school freshmen. The students are ok, but the parents can be a bit of a problem. I don't sleep at all when I have a parent-teacher meeting coming." But her home life is fine. She has been married for 16 years and has two children, age 12 and 8. Both are doing well in school. She loves to cook and to fish. She and her family camp out at least twice a month.

Her past history is totally unremarkable. She doesn't smoke or drink, except for her "hot toddy." She does not take any medications and has no drug allergies. She has never been hospitalized. Her doctor recently did blood tests for thyroid disease and diabetes. She has not had any surgery. Her family history is unremarkable.

The doctor did a thorough examination which was totally normal.

The doctor says, "Normally, I would not do a sleep study for a patient with insomnia but in your circumstance, I think it would be helpful to see exactly how you sleep."

She agrees to have the study which is carried out the following night. She was told to do what she normally does before she goes to bed including the same medications and the "hot toddy."

The sleep study was done. A week later, Rose returns to the office.

The doctor tells her as he shows her the results, "You fell asleep in twenty minutes. Once you were asleep, you stayed asleep without awakenings until about 4 in the morning. They you woke up and dozed off and on until you got out of bed."

"What does it mean?"

"It means we have a difficult problem. You need to completely relearn how to sleep. I would like to send you for Cognitive Behavioral Therapy (CBT) but before you do, I would like to see if we can't help you."

The doctor stopped the Benadryl and "hot toddy." "Both the Benadryl and alcohol really interfere with your sleep." He also told her to stay awake at night until she could not keep her eyes open. "If you get up at 7 AM, you should stay awake until at least 11 PM." He told her to lower the room temperature to 68 degrees and to get rid of the TV. She could take the Ambien, but she was to take it right before she fell asleep. If she wakes up early in the morning, she is to get out of bed and not just lie there.

She agreed to make the changes.

She returned to the doctor two weeks later. "I'm sleeping better. I go to sleep at ten and I get up at 6. I feel good when I get up. I'm more productive at work. My husband says I look better, and I have lost some weight."

The doctor is pleased. He does not think she will need the CBT. "I would like to stop the Ambien. It will be difficult." He gives her a schedule to follow to wean off the Ambien. He will see her in a month.

She does not return.

Background for the presentations

The first case is a classic case of obstructive sleep apnea characterized by severe daytime sleepiness associated with observed episodes of apnea as well as "startles." The metabolic syndrome is associated with sleep apnea in this patient. Likely it occurs because the apnea causes hypoxemia which sets off the inflammatory pathways in large blood vessels. This then causes glucose intolerance which causes the rest of the syndrome including heart disease, hypertension, and even cerebrovascular disease. Sleep apnea can also cause Alzheimer's disease. The second case is a case of mild type 1 narcolepsy. The patient has daytime sleepiness, but she feels good when she gets up in the morning. She has early onset REM sleep but otherwise her sleep study is normal. She also has bizarre dreams when she falls asleep. Her main syndrome is cataplexy or muscle weakness occurring while the patient is alert. Sometimes, the muscle weakness can be quite mild, just involving facial and the muscles of her legs. But sometimes it can be quite severe. Narcolepsy has been described as "an awake brain in a sleeping body." The third patient has insomnia, the most common sleep disorder. In her case, the disorder is mainly due to her lifestyle. Simple changes produced significant benefit.

Important points

1. Sleep apnea is common, but insomnia is much more common.
2. Chronic insomnia is found in 10% of the population!
3. The hallmark symptom of sleep apnea is daytime sleepiness.
4. Sleep apnea occurs more often in obese patients (BMI > 30) and may respond to weight loss.
5. A home sleep study does not measure the AHI (apnea-hypopnea index); rather it measures only respiratory events per hour. Because of this, the severity of sleep apnea may be seriously underreported and worse still, mild cases will be missed. If sleep apnea is suspected and an at home study is negative, a laboratory based sleep study is mandatory.

6. The diagnosis of Narcolepsy requires both a sleep study to exclude sleep apnea as a cause of daytime sleepiness and a multiple sleep latency study to demonstrate daytime sleepiness and early onset REM.
7. The treatment of insomnia is often difficult. Cognitive Behavioral Therapy is the best approach if lifestyle changes fail.
8. The treatment of narcolepsy is directed at both the daytime sleepiness as well as the cataplexy which occurs in about half the patients with narcolepsy.
9. In addition to sleep apnea and narcolepsy, restless leg syndrome can cause daytime sleepiness.

Discussion

You won't find a single soul who doesn't believe that sleep is important for us! But how much sleep do we really need? It depends on how old you are and what type of sleep you are talking about. We have one need for total sleep and one need for rapid eye movement sleep or REM, the type of sleep necessary for learning. Newborns need to sleep about 16 hours a day of which half is REM sleep, while young children sleep about 9 hours a day as REM sleep slowly decreases. An adult requires 7 to 8 hours of sleep of which 20-25% is REM sleep. Every decade after middle age requires about 20 minutes less sleep so that some patients over 70 require between 6 and 6 ½ hours of sleep. Sleeping less than 5 hours or more than 10 hours is associated with illness. After 70, REM accounts for only about 20-25% of sleep time and sleep becomes more and more fragmented.

What determines how much sleep we need? The longer we are awake, the more non-REM sleep we need. The more sleep deprived we are, the longer we will be in delta or Stage 3 non-REM sleep. The more non-REM sleep we have, the more REM sleep we need to get.

Sleep is difficult if the patient has fever or pain or is under stress. Trying to sleep in a room with too much light, especially the blue light of a cell phone, or a lot of noise, or a room that is too hot, will make getting a good night's sleep a challenge. Fatigue interferes with REM sleep. Alcohol makes us sleepy but fragments our sleep. Chemicals such as antihistamines and nicotine have the same effect. Losing or gaining weight also affects sleep. Weight loss leads to more arousals and decreased sleep time, while weight gain increases total sleep time and decreases arousals.

There are several parts of the brain that are important in the sleep-wake cycle. The Reticular Activating System (RAS), located in the upper brainstem, is important in waking us up. If the RAS is diseased, we will sleep forever, even though the cerebral cortex is normal. Between 1915 and 1926 there was an epidemic of "encephalitis lethargica" which affected more than 5 million people. It is a form of encephalitis (inflammation of the brain) commonly referred to as "sleeping sickness." It was first described by the neurologist Constantin von Economo in 1917. It appears to be an autoimmune disease and initially was thought to be related to the great flu epidemic that spanned the world at the time. More recent evidence suggests that the disease was related to Streptococcal pharyngitis. The disease attacks the RAS leaving the patient in a statue-like condition. The patients sit motionless, speechless, totally lacking in initiative, appetite, affect or desire. Whatever happens around them does not affect them in the slightest. One scientist described the patients as ghosts or zombies. About one third of the patients died. None fully recovered.

The hypothalamus also is important in wakefulness. It secretes *hypocretin* which promotes wakefulness, helps maintain motor control, and inhibits REM sleep during wakefulness.

On the other hand, the anterior hypothalamus is involved in making us sleepy. It receives input from the body's "clock," the suprachiasmatic nucleus. The neurotransmitter is Gabapentin, which turns off the centers for wakefulness. If the hypothalamus fails, the patient will stay awake until he drops dead. The condition is called "Fatal Familial Insomnia" which is a prion disease like Mad Cow's Disease. Prions are tiny proteins which cause plaques in the brain. Fatal Familial Insomnia can either be genetic or, less commonly, sporadic. The gene, an autosomal dominant, is found in no more than forty families worldwide. The disease presents in middle age as progressively worsening insomnia, leading to hallucinations, delirium, dementia, and eventually death, usually within eighteen months of the onset of symptoms. The first recorded case was an Italian man, who died in Venice in 1765.

The center for REM sleep is in the Pons. Lesions below the Pons result in EEG findings consistent with REM sleep in the cortex, but no muscle atonia while lesions above the Pons shows no cortical changes of REM sleep but muscle atonia. The neurotransmitter is acetyl choline which "wakes up" the cerebral cortex. If acetyl choline is decreased by damaging the Pons, REM sleep decreases. Acetyl choline analogs injected into the Pons increase REM sleep.

Sleep is divided into two stages, non-REM, and REM sleep. Non-REM sleep is further divided into three stages, stage 1 or light sleep, stage 2, the predominant stage of sleep, and stage 3 or deep sleep. Each stage is characterized by the type of brain waves observed and the clinical state of the patient. In general, there are four types of brain waves. Alpha waves are slightly large and fast. They are generally seen when we are in a light sleep. Beta waves are smaller and faster still. They are found when we are awake or are just a little drowsy. Theta waves are larger and slower waves and are found in stage two sleep. Lastly, Delta waves are the slowest and largest wave. They are seen in deep sleep.

Stage one or light sleep is characterized by the presence of alpha and beta waves. As the person falls into stage one sleep, he or she may experience a sudden generalized muscle jerk which is called a Hypnic Myoclonia. It is totally normal. In stage one, the eyes may show slow rolling movements. There is decreased muscle activity. The heart rate, blood pressure, minute ventilation and cerebral blood flow are all decreased. If the patient is aroused, he will say he has not been sleeping at all even though he may have been snoring!

Stage two is the predominant type of sleep. It accounts almost half of our sleep. The EEG shows slow theta waves which are interrupted by bursts of large waves called sleep spindles and K complexes. These complexes are due to communication between the cerebral cortex and the thalamus or hippocampus. They are likely related to memory and learning. There may also be slow rolling eye motion, or the eyes may be fixed. The muscles are relaxed. The patient is easily arousable, but snoring is often present.

Stage three or deep sleep is characterized by the presence of high amplitude delta waves. The muscles are inactive and there is no eye movement. The pulse rate, blood pressure and respiratory rate are all 30% below awake levels. The patient may dream but the dreams are not bizarre. Bed-wetting and sleepwalking may occur.

REM sleep is a complete contrast to non-REM sleep. The main feature is the presence of rapid eye movement and alpha waves. The EEG appears similar to the EEG of an awake patient! However, all the muscles, except for the diaphragm and the eye muscles are paralyzed. The heart rate and blood pressure increase. During this phase, the patient often has vivid bizarre dreams. The first episode of REM sleep occurs about 90 minutes after falling asleep and recurs about every 90 minutes afterwards. Most of the REM sleep occurs in the second half of sleep.

Throughout the night the patient cycles between the stages of sleep. A graph of the cycling is called a hypnogram. The brain goes from awake to drowsy to Stage 1 NREM, then Stage 2 NREM, then Stage 3 NREM sleep before going to REM. It then recycles another four times during the night, roughly every 90 minutes, until finally the patient awakens, generally, from an episode of REM sleep. The length of the sleep cycle in animals and man is related to the size of the brain.

A **polysomnogram** is a sleep study. It can be done in the sleep laboratory (Level 1 Sleep Study). During the study several parameters are measured including the electroencephalogram (EEG) to determine the level of sleep, the electrooculogram (EOG) to look at eye movements in order to separate non-REM from REM sleep, the electromyogram (EMG) to study muscle tone, the EKG to look at heart rate and the presence of cardiac arrhythmias, and impedance plethysmography (IP) of the chest wall and abdomen to look at respiration in order to determine the presence of air flow as well as movement of the abdominal and chest wall. A nasal flow meter can be used instead to identify air flow. The nasal flow meter cannot measure lung volumes as can a properly calibrated impedance plethysmography system.

A sleep study can also be done at home (Level 3 sleep study). Only a nasal cannula, pulse oximeter, and a device to measure respiratory effort is used. Since an EEG is not done, the AHI (apnea-hypopnea index) cannot be measured—only the number of events occurring over the whole course of the study whether the patient is asleep or awake. Thus, because the patient normally spends 20-30% of the time in bed awake, the frequency of apneas and hypopneas related to actual sleep may be vastly underestimated.

Sleep Disorders

Sleep disorders can be divided into two large groups. The most common disorder is insomnia or the perceived inability to sleep. The second group is those people who are always sleepy.

Insomnia is never a diagnosis. It is a symptom. It is defined as difficulty initiating or maintaining sleep or both. Chronic insomnia, defined by the presence of insomnia three times a week or more for more than three months, affects up to 10% of people but 95% of people report having had at least one episode of insomnia in their life. Chronic insomnia occurs more often in women and its frequency increases as we age. It becomes more common as we grow older, after being widowed or divorced, being in poor health, or having some medical condition such as asthma or COPD. Some medications, especially antidepressants, B-blockers and steroids will make it worse. It is aggravated by over activity and stress. It may be related to mankind's ability to suppress sleep during stress. During 'on-call' nights doctors have disrupted sleep, even if they are not called. Insomnia, even transient insomnia, causes sleep deprivation resulting in daytime fatigue and impaired cognition, both of which can have serious complications.

Transient insomnia is insomnia that *lasts less than two weeks*. It is generally caused by one of three things. It can be due to hyper-alertness, which is related to stress, either good or bad. It can also be due to changing Time Zones or performing Shift Work as in an American couple who fly to Europe or a fireman who has constant changes in his or her work hours. Lastly environmental factors such as loud noises and bright lights can play a role. Of interest, the blue light from our cell phones can even be a cause of transient insomnia.

Persistent insomnia is more of a problem. It is defined as insomnia lasting more than two weeks. It can be caused by problems with the biologic clock or circadian rhythm, hyperthyroidism, hypercorticism including treatment with prednisone, restless leg syndrome, gastroesophageal reflux, fibromyalgia, psychological disease including phobias, anxiety and depression, primary insomnia, or sleep state misperception.

One type of persistent insomnia is due to *Fibromyalgia,* which is a disease of unknown etiology. The symptoms are vague and include muscle pain and weakness associated with tender areas in several parts of the body as well as general fatigue. Insomnia plays a large role in its symptomatology. While these patients have daytime fatigue their sleep latency is normal. The EEG is abnormal with alpha waves superimposed on delta waves.

A second type of persistent insomnia is *Primary Insomnia* which has its onset in childhood. It is a disorder of the brain mechanism that controls sleeping and waking. It is often associated with anxiety and tension. If the onset occurs in later years, the patient may state that he or she sleeps better away from home than at home. Clinically there should be symptoms of both sleep deprivation as well as a prolonged sleep latency.

Persistent insomnia can also be due to *sleep state misperception*. People who suffer from the condition really believe they do not sleep but when they are tested in the sleep lab, their sleep is totally normal. In addition, the multiple sleep latency test is normal indicating no daytime sleepiness. Thus, they believe they are unable to sleep but their "sleeplessness" never affects their daytime functioning.

The key to making the diagnoses in a patient with insomnia is taking a thorough history. A sleep study is rarely indicated or needed. Treatment is directed at the cause and at establishing good sleep hygiene. Medications often have more side effects than benefits.

Daytime hypersomnolence is a "horse of a different color." There are three main causes: sleep apnea, which can be either obstructive sleep apnea or central sleep apnea, narcolepsy, and the restless leg syndrome.

An **apnea** is when we stop breathing. For the apnea to be significant it must be more than 10 seconds long. Patients with **obstructive sleep apnea** stop breathing because their airway becomes blocked. This is almost always due to the anterior pharyngeal wall falling back against the posterior pharyngeal wall during an inspiration. The patient still makes the effort to breathe but just cannot move any air. In contrast people with **central sleep apnea** stop making the effort to breathe. The brain stops sending the signal to the muscles to breathe. There is no respiratory effort at all.

But sometimes the patient doesn't breathe as deeply as normal. A **hypopnea** is defined as an episode of breathing in which the tidal breath is reduced 30% and the oxygen saturation falls at least 4%. A fourth type of sleep disturbance is **respiratory effort related arousals**. These are episodes in which the patient arouses from sleep without meeting the criteria for an apneic or hypopneic event.

Obstructive Sleep Apnea (OSA) is the most common cause of daytime sleepiness. The first description of a patient with the condition was by the writer Charles Dickens in the 19th century in his book *The Pickwick Papers*. He described a young man, a waiter at the Pickwick Club, named "Little Joe" who was extremely obese and suffered from severe daytime sleepiness. Little Joe even fell asleep while standing and knocking on the door of a member of the Pickwick Club.

The hallmark of the disorder is daytime sleepiness associated with significant obstructive apneic events occurring while asleep. The patient or the significant other often reports snoring and startles which are described as "waking up choking." After the patient falls asleep, he will begin having episodes of obstructed breathing. During an episode, air flow will stop, but the patient will continue to move his chest wall and abdominal muscles as if he is gasping for air. After anywhere from ten seconds to a minute and a half, he will suddenly gasp or sit up and gasp. Then, he will lie back down and fall asleep, only to start the cycle over again.

The incidence of mild OSA, an apnea-hypopnea index (AHI) of > 5, is now 20-30% in men and 10-20% in women. If the bar for diagnosing sleep apnea is set at moderate OSA with an AHI of > 15, the incidence is 15% of men and 5% of women. But after a woman passes menopause, she has an equal chance of having OSA.

Patients with obstructive sleep apnea are often obese with a large neck size (greater than 17.5) and a waist size greater than 38. They also tend to be older and more often are men. They may have chronic nasal congestion. Smoking, alcohol abuse, and some classes of medication especially Beta blockers and antihistamines, will worsen the condition. Blacks, Hispanics, and Pacific Islanders are more likely to have obstructive sleep apnea than Caucasians.

The condition is also seen in patients with craniofacial abnormalities such as micrognathia, or in patients with Hypothyroidism, Acromegaly, Down's Syndrome, or large tonsil's (children and patients with HIV). Lastly it can occur in familial aggregations. These patients are often normal in weight and younger than the typical patient.

Surprisingly, Asians have the same incidence of sleep apnea as Americans even though they are much less likely to be overweight. This is most likely due to cranial-facial differences, especially a smaller mid-face.

The first step in making the diagnosis of obstructive sleep apnea is to determine if the patient has daytime sleepiness. The easiest test to use is the Epworth Sleepiness Scale. The patient is asked about the likelihood that he or she will fall asleep during certain activities.

Activity	Score
Sitting and reading	* (0, 1, 2, or 3)
Watching TV	
Sitting inactive in a public place	
Passenger in a car	
Lying down to rest in the afternoon	
Sitting talking to someone	
Sitting after a lunch without alcohol	
In a car stopped in traffic for a few minutes	
TOTAL SCORE (normal is less than 10)	

* Likelihood of falling asleep (0 = never, 1 = slight chance, 2 = moderate chance, 3 = high chance)

If the patient has daytime hypersomnolence then a sleep study should be done. The number of apneas and hypopneas should be measured. Each episode must last 10 seconds. A hypopnea must be associated with a significant fall in tidal volume and oxygen saturation. The sum of the apneas and hypopneas is expressed as the **A-H Index (AHI)** which is simply **the number of apneas and hypopneas per hour of sleep**. Normal is less than 5 per hour; mild sleep apnea is 5-15 per hour; moderate sleep apnea is 15-30 hour; severe obstructive sleep apnea is more than 30 events an hour.

Another study which can be done to evaluate daytime sleepiness is the multiple sleep latency test (MSLT). This test consists of having the patient take five naps at two-hour intervals during the day, often the day following the overnight sleep study. The patient is asked to lie quietly and try to sleep. Each attempt is done for 20 minutes. Sleep latency is the time from lights out to first epoch of sleep lasting more than 15 seconds during a 30 second period. Average latencies of less than five minutes are abnormal. If REM sleep occurs during the MSLT, a condition called narcolepsy is highly likely. We will discuss narcolepsy shortly.

The treatment of obstructive sleep apnea includes the use of positive pressure breathing devices, either CPAP or BIPAP. Both these devices apply positive pressure through the nasal or oral pharynx in order to keep the airway open throughout inspiration and expiration. If that fails to stop the obstruction, a tracheostomy will be curative. Many people do not like having to use the positive pressure device and no one ever wants a tracheostomy. Often the patient will elect to have surgery including radiofrequency ablation of the fatty tissue at the back of the throat or a UPPP (Uvulopalatopharyngoplasty) in which the tonsils and adenoids are removed, and the uvula, soft palate, and pharynx are modified. This less invasive surgery is not effective however. Dental appliances work only for the mildest cases. A newer surgical approach involves electrical stimulation of the hypoglossal nerve. The surgery draws the anterior pharynx anteriorly and opens the airway. A sensor evaluates muscle activity in the chest wall. When activity is noted, a signal is sent to stimulate the hypoglossal nerve to contract and the airway is opened. This type of therapy may one day become standard therapy, but the surgery is quite costly.

The most effective surgery, in more widespread use at the present time, is the maxillary-mandibular advancement which is quite invasive but has an 80-90% success rate.

The long-term effects of untreated sleep apnea are severe and include both *Alzheimer's disease* and the *Metabolic Syndrome*. Sleep apnea is the second most common treatable cause of Alzheimer's disease. The most common treatable cause is hypertension. About half of patients with Alzheimer's disease have sleep-disordered breathing. Sleep apnea causes hypoxemia which damages brain cells. There is a growing body of evidence to support this hypothesis. One study showed that rats exposed for 16 hours a day to decreased O2 levels developed plaques in the brain similar to those of patients with Alzheimer's disease. Another study showed that patients with sleep apnea have "shrunken brain structures" in the part of the brain associated with memory. A third study, using an extremely sensitive MRI study of the brain, showed scattered areas (prefrontal, parietal, and temporal) of brain damage in patients with sleep apnea.

Another complication of sleep apnea is the Metabolic Syndrome. The Metabolic Syndrome is defined as the development of insulin resistance resulting in central obesity, diabetes, hypertension, and hyperlipidemia. It is caused by the release of inflammatory chemicals such as **tumor necrotic factor** from the fatty tissue which causes plaques in arteries of the heart, the brain, and other tissues. Kono et al studied non-obese patients with OSA and found that hyperglycemia and hypertension were more common in patients with OSA than in matched controls and the abnormalities were causally related to the AHI. Another study showed that TIA's and strokes were associated significantly with sleep apnea. Lastly, treatment with CPAP improves insulin sensitivity in patients with OSA. In one study, glucose levels improved significantly after three months of CPAP therapy.

If the metabolic syndrome was not enough, sleep apnea is also associated with depression, suicide, auto accidents, impaired performance at work and even an increased risk of infection due to decreased immune function.

Central sleep apnea is very uncommon. The brain fails to send a signal to the respiratory muscles to contract. It is generally seen in patients who have significantly impaired neurologic disease as well as cardiac disease. These patients develop Cheyne-Stokes respiration, described as a waxing and waning of respiration ending in an apneic episode. Central apnea is also associated with narcotic use and may occur in normal individuals at high altitude. The treatment is to use a non-invasive ventilator such as BIPAP. Neuro-stimulation of the phrenic nerve may become an alternative therapy in the future.

Narcolepsy is an uncommon cause of daytime hypersomnolence. It is defined as *"Sleep-Wake State Instability."* It is an awake brain inside a sleeping body. For an unexplained reason, the physiology of sleep intrudes into wakefulness. Classic Narcolepsy or Type 1 Narcolepsy is characterized not only by daytime sleepiness but also by CATAPLEXY as well as early onset REM sleep. In addition, the patient may describe bizarre hallucinations at the onset of sleep and even sleep paralysis, during which, as the patient begins to fall asleep, he or she becomes unable to move. Patients with Type 2 Narcolepsy do not have cataplexy.

Cataplexy is muscle weakness which occurs whenever the patient becomes excited. It may involve weakness in the facial muscles, a leg or an arm or the patient may just totally collapse. It can last just a few seconds or several minutes.

Narcolepsy can have its onset at any age. The incidence is about 1 in every 2000 people or about 250,000 people world-wide. It is, at least in part, a genetic disease. Animals, including some goats and dachshunds, can be affected.

The diagnosis is made during the sleep study. REM sleep normally does not occur until more than 45 minutes into sleep. In patients with Narcolepsy it may occur immediately upon falling asleep and produce "hypnagogic hallucinations" or night terrors which are severe, vivid nightmares which occur at the onset of sleep. Unlike patients with schizophrenia, patients with narcolepsy do NOT hear voices.

Type 1 Narcolepsy is an auto-immune disorder. The disease attacks the cells of the hypothalamus which produces the chemical hypocretin. Hypocretin increases appetite and produces wakefulness. Hypocretin receptors are found in wake-promoting regions of the brain. Hypocretin levels are immeasurable in the CSF of patients with Type 1 Narcolepsy and hypocretin staining cells are absent in the hypothalamus of narcolepsy patients at autopsy.

Narcolepsy results in poor school and work performance because of daytime sleepiness. In addition, it causes social impairment (avoiding social activities) because of fear of a cataplexic attack. Both these effects lead to isolation and alienation.

The treatment of narcolepsy is at best only fair. Stimulants such as Ritalin or Provigil (Modafenil, which is a pseudo-amphetamine) are used to keep the patient awake. Anti-cataplectic agents including the antidepressants Imipramine and Prozac (SSRI) are also used. The newest and the most effective agent is Zyrem or sodium oxybate which is a central nervous system depressant. It helps prevent cataplexy as well as improve daytime sleepiness.

One simple form of therapy is napping. Napping when tired is also beneficial and should be encouraged in patients with Narcolepsy.

Periodic Leg Movement (PLM) is a common cause of daytime sleepiness. It is characterized by the involuntary twitching or jerking movements occurring while the patient is asleep. It can begin at any age but worsens with aging. Women tend to be more affected than men. While there is some evidence that it may be in part genetic, medications such as Haldol, Reglan, antihistamines, SSRI antidepressants such as Prozac, and alcohol can definitely cause it. It is often associated with the **restless leg syndrome (RSL)**. This syndrome occurs during the day, usually in the evening. The person's legs seem to want to move all the time. Their legs burn or itch. The patient feels like there is something crawling under their skin. If the person tries to keep the legs still, the symptoms get worse. If the patient gets up and moves about, the symptoms are relieved for a short time. About 80% of patients with restless leg syndrome have periodic leg movement disorder. Treatment of the restless leg syndrome is, at best, only fair. The medications commonly used to treat the disease such as Ropinirole and Mirapex can actually cause the disease or make it worse. Gabapentin, opioids such as Codeine and benzodiazepines such as Klonopin may be helpful.

Sleep movement disorders are divided into simple movement disorders such as periodic limb movements, and **Parasomnias,** which include sleepwalking, sleep talking, sleep terrors, and dream enactment. These disorders are much more common in children than adults. Only about one in twenty-five adults suffers from sleep movement disorders whereas up to one in five children are affected. These movement disorders are divided into "simple" and "complex" based on the type of movement and on the underlying type of sleep physiology, whether the movements occur in NREM or REM sleep or in a transition from one stage of sleep to another. The "simple" movement disorders tend to occur when the patient drifts off into sleep or is awakening. The "complex" movements result from a failure of the control mechanism in one of the sleep states.

"Simple" sleep movement disorders include the **hypnic jerk** which occurs at the onset of sleep. They are characterized as a sudden jerk of the entire body. While they are benign, they are quite frightening. **Myoclonus**, or flexion/extension jerks of the abdomen, trunk, or neck is more localized. Like the hypnic jerk, it is benign, generally occurring as the patient is falling asleep. **Nocturnal Leg Cramps** can occur at any time during sleep and, while painful, are also benign. Teeth-grinding or **Bruxism** is another "simple" parasomnia which can result in severe dental injury.

"Complex" movement disorders include classic parasomnias. Sleepwalking is due to NREM sleep and wakefulness becoming intermixed. A sleepwalker will appear to be awake but has minimal cognition and will not remember the event. Most hotels keep robes at the front desk to clothe an unfortunate sufferer of sleepwalking. The staff is instructed to return the poor fellow back to his room without awakening him. **REM sleep behavior disorder (RBD)** occurs when a patient does not have muscle paralysis or atonia which normally occurs during REM sleep. The patient may dream that he is being attacked and fights to defend himself or herself. Normally, during REM sleep the patient's muscles are paralyzed and the patient only dreams he is defending himself but with **RBD** the muscles are not paralyzed, and he can act out the nightmare. In older patients, RBD may be the first sign of dementia, but in younger patients, it is often a sign of narcolepsy.

Suggestions for minor papers

1. Compare narcolepsy and sleep apnea.
2. Why is obstructive sleep apnea more common now?
3. What is meant by "An awake brain in a sleeping body?"
4. What are the causes of central sleep apnea?
5. What is the cause of Cheyne-Stokes respiration?
6. What is restless leg syndrome?

INDEX

"Lung reduction surgery", 11
"sip" ventilation, 126
acetyl choline, 24, 26, 126, 127, 128, 188
acetylcholine receptor, 118
acid fast bacilli, 34, 48
adenocarcinoma, 141, 142
adrenocortical trophic hormone, 137
afterload, 83, 87, 90, 91, 92, 93, 96
air embolism, 58
Alarmin, 27
Alarmins, 22, 27
albumin-cytologic dissociation, 123
Allergic Aspergillosis, 20
allergic bronchopulmonary aspergillosis, 28, 29
Allergic Bronchopulmonary Aspergillosis, 29, 173
Allergic Broncho-Pulmonary Aspergillosis, 175
Allergic Bronchopulmonary Aspergillosis (ABPA), 29
allergic rhinitis, 15
Alpha-1-antitrypsin, 3, 6, 8, 14
Alzheimer's, 104, 107, 125, 186, 193
Amyotrophic Lateral Sclerosis, 115, 120, 121, 124
antidiuretic hormone, 139
anti-proteinases, 8
aortic stenosis, 89, 90, 97
aortic valve stenosis, 87
apoptosis, 141
Arachidonic acid, 28
ARDSNET, 79, 81
asbestos, 110
Asbestosis, 99, 105, 106, 110
Aspergillosis, 15, 20, 168, 169, 175
Aspergillosis fumigatus, 20
Aspergillus, 29
Aspiration, 44
Aspirin Induced Asthma, 28
aTTR gene, 96
atypical Mycobacterium, 13, 166
Bacille Calmette-Guerin, 46
BCG, 46
benralizumab, 27
Berlin Definition, 76
biome, 38, 108
blood clot, 58, 95
blue bloater, 8, 10

BNP, 73, 77, 85, 86, 87, 88, 90, 93, 94, 98
Bondo, 111
brain natriuretic peptide, 93
Bronchial thermoplasty, 28
Bronchiectasis, 1, 7, 13, 173
bronchiectasis., 5, 13, 19, 47, 166, 172
bronchioloalveolar carcinoma, 141
Burkholderia cepacia, 168, 169, 175
cAMP, 171
Campylobacter, 116, 123
Campylobacter gastroenteritis, 116
capillary permeability, 75
cardiac output, 64, 80, 91, 92, 93, 94, 96
cataplexy, 184, 186, 187, 194
Cataplexy, 194
CFTR, 163, 170, 171, 172, 174, 177, 178
check-points, 140
Chlamydia, 38
Chlamydophila pneumoniae, 40
chloride channel, 170, 171, 174
chronic thromboembolic pulmonary hypertension, 66
clubbing, 19, 100, 103, 104, 107, 111, 113, 143, 166, 179
Clubbing, 174
clubbing of the fingers, 143
Coccidioides, 45, 46
Coccidioides immitis, 45, 46
Community acquired pneumonia, 38
Congestive heart failure, 92
continuous positive airway pressure, 36
contractility, 90, 91, 92, 96
COPD assessment test, 12
cor pulmonale, 2, 10, 14, 59, 60, 63, 92, 173
Coronavirus, 37, 41, 72, 73, 74
Covid 19, 37, 42
Covid-19, 42, 43, 123
Covid-19 virus, 42
crepitus, 150, 159
cyclic Adenosine monophosphate, 171
cyclic AMP, 21, 26, 181
cyclic GMP, 21, 24, 26, 66
Cystic Fibrosis, 13, 44, 163, 164, 167, 171, 175, 176, 179
Cystic Fibrosis Foundation, 164, 167, 175
cytokines, 38

D-dimer, 61
Deep vein thrombosis, 58
delayed hypersensitivity, 110
diastolic heart failure, 87, 92
disseminated intravascular coagulation, 77
Dupilumab, 27
echocardiogram, 55, 56, 62, 64, 66, 73, 84, 85, 86, 87, 90, 94, 95, 98, 100, 178
eczema, 15, 16, 20, 22, 24
embolus, 57
empyema, 156
encephalitis lethargica, 187
Endothelin, 65
endothelium, 58
Enterobacter, 44
eosinophil, 12, 16, 19, 20, 23, 27, 29, 30
Epworth Sleepiness Scale, 192
erionite, 161
erythema nodosum, 109
extrinsic allergic alveolitis, 109
extrinsic asthma, 21
Extrinsic asthma, 15, 20
exudate, 154, 157, 158, 161
Factor V, 59, 60
Factor V Leiden, 55, 59, 60, 63
fat embolism, 57, 63, 67, 69, 78
Fat embolism, 63
Fatal familial insomnia, 188
Fatal Familial Insomnia, 188
FeNO, 25
fibrin, 58, 59
fibrinogen, 58
fifty-fifty-fifty club, 9
Flail chest, 153
follicular stimulating hormone, 139
Frank-Starling law, 91
GINA, 25, 30
GINA guidelines, 30
Gold-Bond Sealant, 111
Gram stain, 39, 40, 45, 48, 165
granuloma, 45, 46, 106, 110
granulomas, 46, 103, 108, 109, 112
Guillain-Barré, 115, 121, 123, 124, 126, 127, 131
Hampton Hump, 61
heliox, 36
Hemophilus, 38, 39
hemothorax, 158
heparin, 62
Heparin, 62
HFpEF, 90, 92, 94
HFrEF, 85, 90, 92, 94
Histoplasma, 45, 46

Histoplasma capsulatum, 45, 46
Homan's sign, 53
hospital acquired pneumonia, 44, 48
hydrostatic pressure, 75, 154
hydrothorax, 147
hypercoagulability, 58
Hypersensitivity Pneumonitis, 99, 105, 106, 109
hypertension, 83, 84, 92
hypnagogic hallucinations, 194
Hypnic Myoclonia, 188
hypnogram, 189
hypocretin, 188, 194
hypogammaglobinemia, 13
hypothalamus, 188
immunoglobulin E, 15
Immunoreactive Trypsinogen, 164, 167, 170, 175
influenza, 38, 40, 43
Influenza, 40
insomnia, 188, 189
interferon-gamma release assay, 45
interferon-gamma release assay (IFN-Gamma), 45
Intrinsic asthma, 15, 20
jitter, 118, 127
Kartagener Syndrome, 13
Kerley, 85, 94
Lady Windermere's Syndrome, 6, 13
Lady Wyndemere's Syndrome, 46
large cell carcinomas, 141
Legionella, 38, 40, 48
Legionella pneumophilia, 40
Legionnaire's disease, 40
leukotriene, 15, 21, 27, 28
Löfgren Syndrome, 109
Lovenox, 53, 63, 73, 117, 124
lung protective ventilation, 80, 81, 178
meconium ileus, 173
Meconium ileus, 173, 174
meniscus sign, 156
mepolizumab, 27
mesothelioma, 111, 112, 152, 153, 161
Mesotheliomas, 160
Mestinon, 118, 119, 121, 128
metabolic syndrome, 181, 186
metastasize, 139, 141
methacholine, 24
microbiome, 14, 37, 49, 175
modified Medical Research Council, 12
monoclonal antibodies, 27
MRSA, 39, 44
Mucomist, 176
Multiple Sclerosis, 129, 131
multiple sleep latency test, 184, 192

muscle specific tyrosine kinase, 118
muscle-specific tyrosine kinase, 127
Myasthenia, 121
Myasthenia gravis, 115, 118, 121, 126
Myasthenic Crisis, 121, 128
Mycobacterium avium, 6, 13, 44, 110, 112, 175
Mycobacterium tuberculosis, 44, 45
Mycoplasma, 38, 39, 40
myelin sheath, 115
N-acetycysteine, 176
narcolepsy, 186, 191, 192, 194
Narcolepsy, 181, 184, 186, 187, 194
nasal polyps, 164, 166, 173, 179
nasal potential difference, 170, 175
neprilysin, 96
night terrors, 194
nintedanib, 101, 107, 108
Node of Ranvier, 122, 123
Non-invasive ventilation, 126
Non-Invasive Ventilation, 120
non-REM, 187
non-small cell cancers, 141
Obesity, 29
obstructive sleep apnea, 186
omalizumab, 27
orthopnea, 93
Orthopneumovirus, 40
Oseltamivir, 35
osmotic pressure, 75, 154
Pancoast tumors, 142
pancreas, 163, 170, 171, 172, 173
pancreatitis, 58
pansinusitis, 173
paraneoplasia, 138, 139, 145
parapneumonic effusion, 156
parietal, 147
parietal pleura, 147, 154, 156, 157, 159, 161
paroxysmal nocturnal dyspnea, 93
PCR, 35, 37, 41
percutaneous endoscopic gastrostomy, 115
pericardial effusion, 88
pericardiocentesis, 89
pericarditis, 89, 90, 98
permeability, 69, 75, 76, 78, 154
PET scan, 161
pink puffer, 9, 10
pirfenidone, 101, 107, 108
Platelet, 58
pleural effusion, 45, 111, 144, 147, 153, 154, 155, 156, 157, 158, 160, 161, 162
pleurisy, 31, 38, 60, 142, 156
pleurodesis, 154, 158

Pneumocystis, 45, 47
Pneumocystis jirovecii, 45, 47
pneumothorax, 11, 47, 73, 147, 150, 153, 158, 159, 160, 162, 177
Pneumovax, 48
Poliomyelitis, 115, 131
polymerase chain reaction, 41
polyphonic, 23
polysomnogram, 184, 189
PPD, 33, 34, 45, 46, 89, 100, 137, 138, 139, 145
preload, 90, 91, 92, 93, 95, 96
prion, 188
procalcitonin, 32, 33
prone positioning, 73, 78
Protein C, 59, 60
Protein S, 59
proteinases, 8, 38, 172
prothrombin, 58
pseudobulbar affect, 121
pseudobulbar palsy, 115
Pseudomonas, 44, 49
Pseudomonas aeruginosa, 14, 44, 166, 168
pulmonary artery hypertension, 51, 55, 57
Pulmonary embolism, 57, 59
Pulmonary hypertension, 63, 173
pulmonary infarction, 57, 60
quantitative pilocarpine iontophoresis test (QUIT), 174
racemic epinephrine, 36
reflection coefficient, 75
REM sleep, 187
Remdesivir, 73, 74
renin-angiotensin-aldosterone pathway, 90
reslizumab, 27
respiratory syncytial virus, 36
Respiratory Syncytial Virus, 7, 20, 40
Reticular Activating System, 187
Reverse Transcriptase, 41
Riluzole, 120, 125
RSV vaccine, 36
saddle embolism, 60
Samter's triad, 28
sarcoidosis, 103
Sarcoidosis, 67, 99, 102, 104, 105, 106, 108, 109, 130, 155
Severe Acute Respiratory Syndrome, 41
signet rings, 13, 29, 166
silica, 112
Silicosis, 99, 105, 106, 110, 112
single fiber electromyography, 118
Singular., 27
sleep, 187
sleep latency, 184, 187, 190, 192

sleeping sickness, 187
Small cell carcinoma, 139
Small cell lung cancers, 141
spelunkers, 47
Spironolactone, 85
Squamous cell carcinoma, 139
Squamous cell carcinomas, 141
Starling's law, 75
stomata, 147, 154
Streptococcus, 33, 37, 38, 39
Streptococcus pneumoniae, 33, 37, 38, 39, 165
stroke volume, 91, 92
surface tension, 75
surfactant, 75, 76, 141
Swan-Ganz catheter, 71, 73, 95, 159
sweat test, 5, 16, 19, 20, 164, 166, 167, 170, 174, 175
systolic heart failure, 92
Tamiflu, 35, 44, 72
Tezepelumab, 27
The Global Initiative for Obstructive Lung Disease, 12
thermoplasty, 28
thoracentesis, 149, 152, 157
thrombin, 58
thromboembolic pulmonary hypertension, 57, 64, 66
thrombus, 58, 59
thymic stromal lymphopoietin, 22
Thymic stromal lymphopoietin, 21
Thymoma, 128
thymus gland, 118, 128
tobramycin, 170, 176
toluene diisocyanate, 15, 19
tram-lines, 7, 13, 19
trans-catheter aortic valve replacement, 87
transudate, 154, 155, 157
trepopnea, 156
Trepopnea, 156
TSLP, 22, 27
tuberculosis, 5, 6, 13, 28, 31, 34, 45, 46, 88, 89, 92, 97, 98, 108, 112, 137, 138, 149, 155, 156, 157, 158, 166
Usual Interstitial Pneumonitis, 99, 100, 105, 106
Velcro Rales, 107
Vericiguat, 97
Virchow's triad, 57
Virchow's Triad, 58
visceral, 147
visceral pleura, 147, 158
Voriconazole, 169
Wegener's Granulomatosis, 99, 106
Well's criteria, 61
Zyrem, 194

muscle specific tyrosine kinase, 118
muscle-specific tyrosine kinase, 127
Myasthenia, 121
Myasthenia gravis, 115, 118, 121, 126
Myasthenic Crisis, 121, 128
Mycobacterium avium, 6, 13, 44, 110, 112, 175
Mycobacterium tuberculosis, 44, 45
Mycoplasma, 38, 39, 40
myelin sheath, 115
N-acetycsteine, 176
narcolepsy, 186, 191, 192, 194
Narcolepsy, 181, 184, 186, 187, 194
nasal polyps, 164, 166, 173, 179
nasal potential difference, 170, 175
neprilysin, 96
night terrors, 194
nintedanib, 101, 107, 108
Node of Ranvier, 122, 123
Non-invasive ventilation, 126
Non-Invasive Ventilation, 120
non-REM, 187
non-small cell cancers, 141
Obesity, 29
obstructive sleep apnea, 186
omalizumab, 27
orthopnea, 93
Orthopneumovirus, 40
Oseltamivir, 35
osmotic pressure, 75, 154
Pancoast tumors, 142
pancreas, 163, 170, 171, 172, 173
pancreatitis, 58
pansinusitis, 173
paraneoplasia, 138, 139, 145
parapneumonic effusion, 156
parietal, 147
parietal pleura, 147, 154, 156, 157, 159, 161
paroxysmal nocturnal dyspnea, 93
PCR, 35, 37, 41
percutaneous endoscopic gastrostomy, 115
pericardial effusion, 88
pericardiocentesis, 89
pericarditis, 89, 90, 98
permeability, 69, 75, 76, 78, 154
PET scan, 161
pink puffer, 9, 10
pirfenidone, 101, 107, 108
Platelet, 58
pleural effusion, 45, 111, 144, 147, 153, 154, 155, 156, 157, 158, 160, 161, 162
pleurisy, 31, 38, 60, 142, 156
pleurodesis, 154, 158

Pneumocystis, 45, 47
Pneumocystis jirovecii, 45, 47
pneumothorax, 11, 47, 73, 147, 150, 153, 158, 159, 160, 162, 177
Pneumovax, 48
Poliomyelitis, 115, 131
polymerase chain reaction, 41
polyphonic, 23
polysomnogram, 184, 189
PPD, 33, 34, 45, 46, 89, 100, 137, 138, 139, 145
preload, 90, 91, 92, 93, 95, 96
prion, 188
procalcitonin, 32, 33
prone positioning, 73, 78
Protein C, 59, 60
Protein S, 59
proteinases, 8, 38, 172
prothrombin, 58
pseudobulbar affect, 121
pseudobulbar palsy, 115
Pseudomonas, 44, 49
Pseudomonas aeruginosa, 14, 44, 166, 168
pulmonary artery hypertension, 51, 55, 57
Pulmonary embolism, 57, 59
Pulmonary hypertension, 63, 173
pulmonary infarction, 57, 60
quantitative pilocarpine iontophoresis test (QUIT), 174
racemic epinephrine, 36
reflection coefficient, 75
REM sleep, 187
Remdesivir, 73, 74
renin-angiotensin-aldosterone pathway, 90
reslizumab, 27
respiratory syncytial virus, 36
Respiratory Syncytial Virus, 7, 20, 40
Reticular Activating System, 187
Reverse Transcriptase, 41
Riluzole, 120, 125
RSV vaccine, 36
saddle embolism, 60
Samter's triad, 28
sarcoidosis, 103
Sarcoidosis, 67, 99, 102, 104, 105, 106, 108, 109, 130, 155
Severe Acute Respiratory Syndrome, 41
signet rings, 13, 29, 166
silica, 112
Silicosis, 99, 105, 106, 110, 112
single fiber electromyography, 118
Singular., 27
sleep, 187
sleep latency, 184, 187, 190, 192

sleeping sickness, 187
Small cell carcinoma, 139
Small cell lung cancers, 141
spelunkers, 47
Spironolactone, 85
Squamous cell carcinoma, 139
Squamous cell carcinomas, 141
Starling's law, 75
stomata, 147, 154
Streptococcus, 33, 37, 38, 39
Streptococcus pneumoniae, 33, 37, 38, 39, 165
stroke volume, 91, 92
surface tension, 75
surfactant, 75, 76, 141
Swan-Ganz catheter, 71, 73, 95, 159
sweat test, 5, 16, 19, 20, 164, 166, 167, 170, 174, 175
systolic heart failure, 92
Tamiflu, 35, 44, 72
Tezepelumab, 27
The Global Initiative for Obstructive Lung Disease, 12
thermoplasty, 28
thoracentesis, 149, 152, 157
thrombin, 58
thromboembolic pulmonary hypertension, 57, 64, 66
thrombus, 58, 59
thymic stromal lymphopoietin, 22
Thymic stromal lymphopoietin, 21
Thymoma, 128
thymus gland, 118, 128
tobramycin, 170, 176
toluene diisocyanate, 15, 19
tram-lines, 7, 13, 19
trans-catheter aortic valve replacement, 87
transudate, 154, 155, 157
trepopnea, 156
Trepopnea, 156
TSLP, 22, 27
tuberculosis, 5, 6, 13, 28, 31, 34, 45, 46, 88, 89, 92, 97, 98, 108, 112, 137, 138, 149, 155, 156, 157, 158, 166
Usual Interstitial Pneumonitis, 99, 100, 105, 106
Velcro Rales, 107
Vericiguat, 97
Virchow's triad, 57
Virchow's Triad, 58
visceral, 147
visceral pleura, 147, 158
Voriconazole, 169
Wegener's Granulomatosis, 99, 106
Well's criteria, 61
Zyrem, 194

www.ingramcontent.com/pod-product-compliance
Lightning Source LLC
Chambersburg PA
CBHW080957170526
45158CB00010B/2827